Penguin Books

Penguin Nursing Revi
OPHTHALMIC N

Other titles in this series:

Care for the Elderly
Ear, Nose and Throat Nursing
General Medical Nursing
Orthopaedic Nursing
Principles of Nursing
Surgical Nursing

Penguin Nursing Revision Notes
Advisory Editor: P. A. Downie

■ Ophthalmic Nursing

Revised edition

Penguin Books

PENGUIN BOOKS

Published by the Penguin Group
27 Wrights Lane, London W 8 5 T Z, England
Viking Penguin Inc., 40 West 23rd Street, New York, New York 10010, U S A
Penguin Books Australia Ltd, Ringwood, Victoria, Australia
Penguin Books Canada Ltd, 2801 John Street, Markham, Ontario, Canada L 3 R 1 B 4
Penguin Books (N Z) Ltd, 182–190 Wairau Road, Auckland 10, New Zealand

Penguin Books Ltd, Registered Offices: Harmondsworth, Middlesex, England

This revised edition first published in Penguin Books 1989
10 9 8 7 6 5 4 3 2 1

Made and printed in Great Britain by
Cox and Wyman Ltd, Reading, Berks.
Typeset in 9/10½ pt Linotron 202 Galliard by
Rowland Phototypesetting Ltd, Bury St Edmunds, Suffolk

Contents

Advisory editor's note

This series of revision aids first saw the light of day in the early 1980s and has been reprinted numerous times thus indicating that the books fulfil a real need. Now they have been revised and updated. Many nurses, both tutors and ward sisters, have helped and advised in these revisions; they are too numerous to list individually but the warm thanks of the publishers and the advisory editor are extended to each of them.

These small books are not textbooks, *but* revision aids; consequently they aim to indicate principles and outlines rather than in-depth descriptions. Where specific treatments and care are discussed the reader should remember that they are not necessarily the only methods. All hospitals have their own laid-down treatment procedures and protocols and nurses must always apprise themselves of these.

Clinical terminology has been used throughout, though where there is an anatomical or scientific term this is shown also, and both terms are used simultaneously.

Care plans are shown in some of the books, but all the books lay emphasis on the four parts of the nursing process which can be turned into effective care plans, namely assessment, planning, implementation and evaluation. *Care* for patients is the *raison d'être* of all nursing and while these books are essentially revision aids for examinations, they nevertheless emphasize the nurse's role in the direct care of the patient.

Examinations might be described as 'necessary evils' in that they provide a means of ensuring that a person has reached an acceptable standard of competence. These books are intended as aids to help attain this standard; essentially they are for learners rather than nurses undergoing post-basic courses. Suggestions to help both study and the actual examination are included as is a short list of relevant reading. Specific references have not been included but learners are advised to make full use of their School of Nursing library and to seek help in learning how to seek out references from the librarian and their tutors.

In the 1850s, Florence Nightingale discussing how to teach nurses to nurse wrote in her *Notes on Nursing*, 'I do not pretend to teach her how, I ask her to teach herself, and for this purpose I venture to give her some hints.' Now, some hundred years on it falls to Penguin Books Limited to offer 'some hints' to the learner nurse of the present day as she prepares for her examinations.

P.D.
Norwich 1988

Introduction

■ THE CONTEXT OF OPHTHALMIC NURSING – SOME IMPORTANT CONSIDERATIONS

Ophthalmic nursing has developed rapidly during recent years and changes reflect developments in the following areas:

1 New demands for health care in a changing society.
2 Advances in technology and microsurgery.
3 Developments within the nursing profession itself.

Each of these has contributed to a changing emphasis in patient care. The result of these factors has been that many more people receive care on an outpatient basis, and episodes of hospitalization are, in general, short. Currently we are seeing an emergence of day-case surgery throughout the United Kingdom.

This situation provides the nurse with a challenge in health care. Given the increasing outpatient commitment and the short length of hospital stay, it is imperative that emphasis is placed on an individualized approach to care. Many departments have turned their attention to carrying out a comprehensive assessment of the needs of a patient attending the outpatient department, prior to hospital admission. In this way the patient's needs can be anticipated, and where problems may occur as a result of early discharge from hospital, these can be identified at an early stage and care planned appropriately with community support, as necessary. This approach also enhances continuity of care.

Many people attend the ophthalmic department; for some it will be a visit to the accident and emergency department, and only a few visits will be required. For others it may be the start of regular outpatient appointments; with the increase in this aspect of care more demands are placed upon the nurse who, having assessed the needs of the individual patient, will be required to teach and advise if compliance with treatment is to be achieved effectively.

For many people attendance in the ophthalmic department may mean that they become aware that their sight is going to deteriorate, but whatever the reason for attending, the patient will be apprehensive and will look to the nursing and medical staff for sensitive reassurance.

Most patients will be elderly and some may have other disabilities, so time should be allowed for helping the patient to-and-from the doctor, for the patient to absorb the information given, and for an opportunity to ask questions. Nursing evaluation of his understanding will be important if he is to feel secure, and able to participate in his own care.

Periods of admission to hospital may be unsettling. The patient may fear that the surgery or medical treatment will not be successful. If the patient has previously led an active life he may experience difficulty in coming to terms with temporary or permanent visual disability, whatever the degree of this disability.

Listening to and talking with a patient play a major part in ophthalmic nursing care. During hospitalization the patient may welcome the provision of a radio with earphones, or a Talking Book.

Patient safety is an essential consideration and the nurse should ensure that there are no obstacles in the ward or department, such as trailing flexes or medical machinery, and that bed castors are turned inwards. The patient should have ease of access to the nurse-call system and his general comfort should be ensured within the context of self-care appropriate in current ophthalmic nursing practice.

Pre-operatively the nurse should explain to the patient what will be involved in his preparation for surgery, his anaesthetic (whether local or general) and operative procedure, and what to expect following surgery. The importance of adequate pre-operative preparation and its significance for postoperative recovery has been stressed in studies such as Boore (1979).

Ophthalmic nursing, in its current development, is both challenging and rewarding; it requires of the nurse sensitivity, founded on a broad knowledge base, and the acquisition of precise nursing skills. It provides scope for health education, patient teaching and nursing research and, as it progresses, extension of the nurse's role within acceptable professional guidelines.

Within the text examples of commonly used ophthalmic drugs have been given but it should be remembered that each hospital will be variable in prescribing.

■ REFERENCE

Boore, J. (1979). *Prescription for Recovery*. Royal College of Nursing, London.

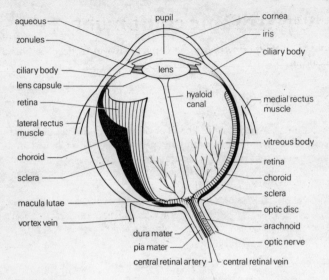

Fig. 1 The eyeball

Labels for Fig. 1:
aqueous
zonules
ciliary body
lens capsule
retina
lateral rectus muscle
choroid
sclera
macula lutae
vortex vein
pupil
lens
hyaloid canal
dura mater
pia mater
central retinal artery
cornea
iris
ciliary body
medial rectus muscle
vitreous body
retina
choroid
sclera
optic disc
arachnoid
optic nerve
central retinal vein

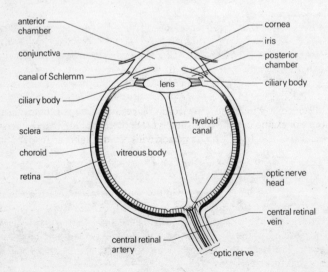

Fig. 2 The eyeball

Labels for Fig. 2:
anterior chamber
conjunctiva
canal of Schlemm
ciliary body
sclera
choroid
retina
vitreous body
lens
hyaloid canal
central retinal artery
optic nerve
cornea
iris
posterior chamber
ciliary body
optic nerve head
central retinal vein

1 Ophthalmic equipment

■ THE ROOM

The examination room should be of an adequate size to allow the patient and the relevant staff comfort and privacy.

The floor should be clear of any trailing wires to ensure patient safety. It must be possible to block out light from the room – this is essential for some types of ocular examination.

Ideally, the room should be at least 6 metres long to accommodate a Snellen's test type for estimation of visual acuity, or 3 metres long to accommodate a reverse test type.

■ SNELLEN'S TEST TYPE (Fig. 3)

This is a flat wall-mounted chart, or four-sided illuminated box. The chart consists of a series of letters graduated in size and arranged in horizontal rows. The top row consists of one letter, and as the patient reads down the rows the letters become correspondingly smaller. Each line is expressed as a fraction; the top letter is designed to be used at 60 metres (m), and the subsequent rows at 36, 24, 18, 12, 9, 6 and 5 metres. A person with normal vision can read the seventh line at 6m, and his visual acuity is recorded as 6/6. The upper number indicates the distance that the patient is from the chart, i.e. in the case above 6m, and the lower number indicates the distance at which the letter could be read by a person with normal vision. For example, if the recording is 6/18, this illustrates that the person can read at 6m the letter which a person with normal sight can read at 18m.

■ To record visual acuity

The patient should be seated comfortably and an assessment of his understanding of the procedure ascertained. An explanation of the procedure should be made suitable to the individual.

The patient is asked to cover one eye and to read as far down the chart as he is able. The result of this is recorded in his notes; the visual acuity of the other eye is then similarly tested.

If the patient wears distance glasses or contact lenses, the visual acuity is

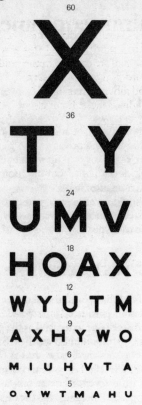

Fig. 3 A Snellen's test type

recorded in the same way, with refraction. In this case a note should be added to the recording to indicate that the patient was wearing glasses or contact lenses during the test.

If the patient is unable to see 6/60, he is given a *pin-hole* – a black disc with a tiny hole at its centre, the purpose being to establish a measurement of central vision. He is asked to cover one eye, to hold the pin-hole to the other and to focus on the letters through the pin-hole. The result is recorded as above, with reference to the use of a pin-hole.

If the patient cannot see 6/60 he is asked to move forward, a metre at a time, and if any of the letters are read, these are recorded, e.g. the top letter at half the distance would be recorded as 3/60.

If the patient cannot see at a reduced distance he is asked to sit down again, to cover one eye at a time and the nurse will hold up several fingers. The patient is asked to count them and this is recorded as *CF – count fingers*. Failing this the eyes are covered in turn and a hand waved in front of the eye. This is recorded as *hand movements*.

If he cannot see hand movements a light is shone towards each eye to see if PL (perception of light) is there. If not, this will be recorded as 'no PL'.

As an alternative to letters on the test type cards, 'E' Charts, numbers and animals are available.

■ The 'E' Chart

The Es on the test type are graded in the same manner and the patient holds a cardboard 'E' and turns it to the same position as those on the chart. Numbers and animals are suitable for children or patients unable to read and are recorded in the same way as the letter chart.

■ READING TESTS FOR NEAR VISION

These are tests to establish how well the patient can see to read at close range. The one most commonly used is the N series. The patient is seated by a good light. He is handed a booklet which contains several typeset paragraphs each headed by a letter and number. The smallest type is N5 and as each number increases the typeset becomes larger. The numbers start at N5 and continue to N48. A patient considered to have normal vision should read N6. Each eye is checked as in Snellen's distance testing and both eyes are recorded. The letter and number of the paragraphs are entered into the patient's notes. These are recorded with and without reading glasses.

■ THE DIRECT OPHTHALMOSCOPE

This is a hand instrument powered by batteries or electricity via a transformer and made up of a head and handle. The handle contains the power source. The head is made up of a perforated mirror, a series of lenses and a tiny light.

a The doctor usually examines the eyes with the patient seated looking straight ahead, the non-affected eye first, then the affected eye. The patient is then asked to direct the gaze as requested by the doctor.

b The eyes may be examined through the natural pupil or through a dilated pupil. This depends on the patient's condition and the doctor's wishes. If the doctor asks for one or both eyes to be dilated a mydriatic such as Mydrilate 0.5% or 1% may be used as this gives a quick mydriasis and is reversible. Before instilling a mydriatic the nurse should check if the patient has glaucoma. The patient should be warned that he will have blurred vision following instillation of drops. The patient should be reminded again about the blurred vision and preferably should be accompanied to any other department being visited. Car drivers and machinery operators should also be reminded about the dangers of operating vehicles or machinery while blurred vision remains.

Through the ophthalmoscope the doctor will be able to see the structures to the back of the eye and may be able to detect some ocular defects.

■ SPECTACLES AND LENSES

Refraction may be defined as (1) the deviation in the course of rays of light in passing from one transparent medium into another of different density: or (2) the determination of refractive errors of the eye, and their correction by glasses. During refraction (testing a person's eyesight) it is necessary to use a trial frame and lenses. The trial frame is a spectacle-shaped piece of apparatus which the patient wears as if it were a pair of spectacles. It has three functions:

 a measuring interocular diameter
 b adjusting bridge height
 c angling of frame to face.

Each eye-piece on the trial frame has three slots into which the lenses are placed to check the refraction. On the outer part degrees are marked from 0° to 180° in 10-degree divisions and in between the 5° are marked by a dot. The degrees are marked to determine the axis of cylindrical lenses. When the cylindrical lenses are placed in the trial frame they can be rotated to obtain maximum vision and then the angle where that degree of vision is obtained is recorded and also the strength of the lens.

The lenses are small round discs of glass. In a lens box two of each strength lens are supplied ranging from +0.05 to +20 dioptres (a unit of measurement of strength of the refractive power of lenses or prisms) and from −0.05 to −20 dioptres. Their strength is recorded in dioptres. The plus lenses are convex and the minus lenses are concave. Each glass lens is encased in a small metal or plastic circle on which the strength is marked, + in red and − in black. Great care should be taken in handling the lenses, always holding them on the outer edges and they should be polished on a regular basis to keep them free from smears, dirt and scratches.

Also contained in the box are:
1 convex and concave spheres
2 convex and concave cylinders
3 prisms
4 pin-hole
5 slit aperture
6 cross cylinder
7 red disc
8 green disc
9 Maddox rod.

■ ISHIHARA CHARTS

This is a test for colour vision. It is a box of coloured printed plates in which different numbers are printed in spots of colour on a background of confusion colours.

■ TRANSILLUMINATOR

This is an instrument shaped like a pencil torch with a beam of light on one end. If a tumour of the eye is suspected, transillumination is performed. Both eyes should be dilated with mydriatics. The eye is examined by projecting the beam of light through the eyelid towards the globe or by using local anaesthetic drops, e.g. amethocaine 1% to render the eye insensitive. The transilluminator is then placed on the conjunctiva and the glow of light is seen through the pupil and transilluminates through the globe. If there is a solid structure (tumour) through which the light fails to pass, no glow will be seen. The result is recorded on the notes.

■ SLIT LAMP

The slit lamp is a combination of binocular microscope and slit lamp which is extensively used to provide detailed examination of the anterior segment of the eye. With some extra attachments, the posterior segment including retina and optic disc can be examined.

The patient sits on a chair or stool with the chin placed on a chin rest and the forehead resting against a head bar. The patient is asked to look straight ahead, not at the light. The doctor sits on the opposite side facing the patient and looks through the microscope. By the use of magnification and lighting, the correct focus can be obtained and by the movement of a stick attached to the instrument the anterior segment of the eye can be examined fully. Several attachments are used.

■ Applanator for tonometry

This records the patient's intra-ocular tension. Normal tension limits on the applanator are 15–22mmHg. (Hg = mercury.)

■ Gonioscope

This is a contact lens, placed on the anterior part of the eye, after the cornea and conjunctiva have been anaesthetized. Once it is in place the lens shows the angle in the anterior chamber in greater detail.

■ Three-mirror contact lens

The eye is anaesthetized and the contact lens inserted: this three-mirror lens will show for examination the whole of the fundus, the angle of the anterior chamber and the ciliary body.

■ Hruby lens

This lens is attached to the head rest of the slit lamp and sits in front of the patient's eye. This allows binocular magnified examination of the vitreous humour and retina.

■ Fundus contact lens

This is inserted into the eye after it has been anaesthetized and will give the same view as the Hruby lens.

■ VISUAL FIELD TESTS

The field of vision may be defined as central and peripheral.

■ Central field test using a Bjerrum screen

a To detect any defect of the central field within a radius of 30°.
b To estimate the size of the blind spot.
The Bjerrum screen is a thick black piece of fabric measuring one metre square and suspended on a frame. A circle in white is printed on the fabric and four other circles are printed within the main circle at equal distances.

At the very centre of the circle is a white spot, with lines drawn at every 15° from the white dot to the outer circle.

The patient is seated 1 metre from the screen, the room darkened and a strong light behind the patient directed on to the screen. A black rod is used with a 1mm or 2mm white disc attached to the end of the rod. The procedure is explained to the patient and one eye is covered. With the uncovered eye the patient fixes on the white spot in the centre of the circle. The rod is brought slowly from the outside of a circle with the white disc towards the patient and the patient is asked to communicate when he sees the white disc in his field of vision. At the beginning of each field test the size of the blind spot (head of the optic nerve) is determined using a 10mm white disc. All chartings on the screen are done using black-headed pins. The movement of the rod is repeated all the way round the field using the markings on the screen. At the end of the field the patient rests while the pin markings on the screen are transferred on to a printed chart which will have the patient's name, size of disc used, hopital number, correct eye and date of test on it. If both eyes are to be tested the procedure is repeated using the other eye, and the result transferred on to a separate chart with the above details written on it.

Patients having this test performed for the first time may find it difficult to begin with but patients who have their fields checked at regular intervals become very competent.

Where colour fields are requested the same procedure is carried out using a coloured disc on the rod, e.g. red, blue and green. Each result is charted stating which colour disc was used.

Where the patient is unable to see a 1 or 2mm disc, a larger disc should be used. They are supplied in packs up to 10mm. Each disc increases in size by 1mm.

■ Reasons for recording central fields

1 Glaucoma.
2 Diseases of central nervous system, e.g. tumours, aneurysm, haemor-rhage.

■ Peripheral fields tests

□ *Confrontation test*

The patient is seated with his back to the light and asked to close his left eye. The doctor is seated in front of the patient and at the same height (it must be taken that the doctor has normal fields). The doctor closes his right eye and with his arm and fingers extended between himself and the patient he moves his hand from different points of the periphery inwards.

The patient is asked to communicate when he sees the movement of the fingers.

□ *Perimetry*

This is a more accurate method but takes a little longer than the confrontation method.

The instrument consists of an arc which can be revolved. The arc is marked in degrees: 0° is in the middle and 90° to each outer part. The patient sits with his chin on a chin rest and one eye is covered. The uncovered eye fixes on an illuminated cross at the centre of the arc. A beam of light is brought in from the end of the arc to the centre and the patient is asked to communicate when he sees the beam. A chart is placed on the instrument (marked in degrees) and the operator records straight on to the chart. The chart should be labelled as for central fields. If both eyes are to be recorded, the procedure is repeated making sure that the second eye is level with the illuminated cross on the centre of the arc.

□ *Reasons for recording peripheral fields*

1 Glaucoma.
2 Diseases of the central nervous system.
3 Pigmentary degeneration of the retina.

■ INDIRECT OPHTHALMOSCOPE

The binocular indirect ophthalmoscope is worn on the head, using a plastic adjustable head frame. On the front is a light and reflecting mirrors. The light is reflected through a +20 or +30 dioptre convex lens through the patient's pupil and a stereoscopic view of the fundus is seen. Prior to this examination the doctor will ask for the patient's pupils to be dilated and drops used may be Mydrilate 1% or homatropine 1%. These drops are instilled until dilation is achieved.

■ Reasons for using indirect ophthalmoscope

1 Retinal detachment, surgery of retina and other retinal disorders.
2 Intra-ocular tumours.

■ PRACTICE QUESTIONS

1 Name the test type used for checking distance vision.
2 Name the test type used for checking near vision.

3 What length should the room be to accommodate a Snellen's test type?

4 List the fractions in which 6-metre vision is recorded.

5 If patients cannot read 6/60 on the test type what other methods are employed to record their vision?

6 What alternatives to letters are available on the test type cards?

7 Name the two types of ophthalmoscope used in ophthalmology.

8 Name one common mydriatic drop used to dilate the pupil prior to examination.

9 What effect does a mydriatic have upon the patient's vision?

10 What should a patient who has had a mydriatic drop instilled be warned against when leaving the hospital department?

11 Name the three functions of the trial frame.

12 What two types of spheres are contained in the lens box?

13 Name the two types of cylinders in the lens box.

14 Give five names of accessories in the lens box.

15 What do you understand by the term Ishihara charts?

16 What function does the transilluminator have?

17 What attachments are available for the slit lamp?

18 What two fields' tests are performed?

19 What is the name of the screen used in the central field test?

20 Give the reasons for recording central fields.

21 Name the two types of peripheral field tests.

22 Give the reasons for recording peripheral fields.

23 What are the reasons for using the **indirect** ophthalmoscope?

24 What structures of the eye will be seen when looking through the **direct** ophthalmoscope?

■ Answers

1 Snellen's test type

2 'N' series

3 6 metres or 3 metres for a reverse test type.

4 6/60, 6/36, 6/24, 6/18, 6/12, 6/9, 6/6, 6/5, 6/4.

5 Use pin-hole, try 3-metre distance, counting fingers or hand movements, numbers and animals.

6 'E' chart, numbers and animals.

7 Direct and indirect.

8 Mydrilate eyedrops 0.5% or 1%.

9 Causes blurring of vision.

10 The patient should be reminded about blurred vision; car drivers and machinery operators should also be reminded about operating such appliances while blurred vision remains.

11   Measures interocular diameter, adjusts bridge height and helps in angling of frame to face.

12   Concave and convex.

13   Concave and convex.

14   Concave and convex spheres, concave and convex cylinders, prisms, pin-holes, slit aperture, cross cylinder, red disc, green disc, Maddox rod.

15   A test for colour vision. It is a box of coloured printed plates in which different numbers are printed in spots of colour on a background of confusion colours.

16   To detect through a dilated pupil the presence of a growth (tumour).

17   Applanator for tonometry, gonioscope, 3-mirror contact lens, Hruby lens, fundus contact lens.

18   Central and peripheral.

19   Bjerrum.

20   Glaucoma, diseases of central nervous system (CNS), tumours, aneurysm and haemorrhage.

21   Confrontation and perimetry.

22   Glaucoma; diseases of central nervous system (CNS); pigmentary degeneration of the retina.

23   Retinal detachment and surgery of retina; intra-ocular tumours.

24   Through the ophthalmoscope the doctor will be able to see the structures to the back of the eye and be able to pick up any defect in the conjunctiva, cornea, anterior chamber, iris, pupil, lens, vitreous, and retina.

2 Nursing procedures within the ophthalmic department

The nursing procedures described in this chapter are all carried out in the ward or the outpatient department. It should be remembered that they should be carried out with an individual approach to care.

Many people are understandably fearful of having 'something done to their eyes', and some people attending the department will be blind or partially sighted, so a gentle approach and an awareness of the problems associated with temporary or permanent visual loss are always needed.

In many ophthalmic outpatient departments, a prescription for eye-drops will be written in the patient's outpatient notes, rather than on the general medical chart. If this is the case, the responsible nurse must check the medication accurately from the patient's notes and ensure that the correct patient is identified for administration of the prescribed drops.

■ THE EYELIDS

The eyelids are movable folds of tissue, the functions of which are:
1 To protect the eye from external injury, foreign body, over-exposure, excess light.
2 To assist in the lubrication of the eye; tears are secreted from lacrimal glands and the lids help to pass the tear film over the front of the eye to keep the cornea moist.
3 To cleanse any dust which may be in the conjunctival sac by the action of blinking.

The eyelids consist of:
1 *Skin*: The thinnest in the body, it is loose and elastic, permitting extreme swelling in the case of trauma or inflammation.
2 *Tarsal plates*: These consist of fibrous and elastic tissue.
3 *Conjunctiva*: This lines the tarsal plates, and provides a smooth surface over the front of the eye. The conjunctiva which lines the lids is known as *the palpebral conjunctiva*.
4 *Muscles*:
   a The orbicularis oculi muscle which receives its innervation from the facial (7th cranial) nerve is roughly circular. Its function is to close the lids.

b The levator palpebrae muscle receives its innervation from the oculo-motor (3rd cranial) nerve. Its function is to elevate the upper lid.

■ **The glands of the eyelids**

There are four types of glands in the eyelids: meibomian glands; the glands of Moll; and Zeis; and the accessory lacrimal glands (of Krause and Wolfring).

The meibomian glands are long sebaceous glands in the tarsal plate. These glands do not communicate with the hair follicles. There are about 25 in the upper lid, and 20 in the lower lid. The meibomian glands produce a sebaceous substance that forms an oily layer on the surface of the tear film. The function of this is to prevent a rapid evaporation of the normal tear layer.

The glands of Zeis are modified sebaceous glands.

The glands of Moll are sweat glands.

The accessory lacrimal glands (Krause and Wolfring) supply moisture to the conjunctival sac and the cornea.

■ **Blood supply**

This is delivered from the following arteries:
ophthalmic
facial
superficial temporal
infra-orbital.

Drainage is via the following veins:
ophthalmic
temporal
facial.

■ **Lymphatics**

Lymph drains to the pre-auricular, parotid and sub-maxillary lymph nodes.

■ **Nerves**

Oculomotor (3rd cranial) nerve.
Facial (7th cranial) nerve.
Sensory nerve supply is from the trigeminal (5th cranial) nerve via the ophthalmic and maxillary branches.

■ **Eyelashes**

The lashes are short thick curved hairs. Their roots are embedded into the connective tissue and muscle.

■ THE LACRIMAL APPARATUS (Fig. 4)

Two lacrimal glands are situated on the upper and outer aspect of orbit in a depression in the frontal bone.

The glands are about the size of an almond. There are approximately 12 ducts which conduct tears to the upper and outer aspect of the eyeball.

■ TEARS

Constituents:
water
salts
lysozyme – anti-bacterial function.

Tears drain into the puncta then through the puncta into the lacrimal canaliculus, upper and lower. There are two of these, one in each eyelid. These tiny channels drain into the lacrimal sac. The lacrimal sac is situated in a fossa in the lacrimal bone – upper expanded parts of the nasolacrimal

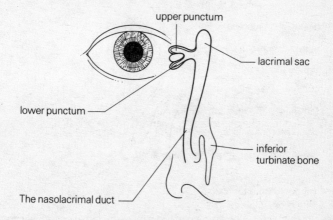

Fig. 4 Lacrimal apparatus

duct. This duct is approximately 2cm in length and opens into the nasal cavity, a membranous canal which opens into the nose at the level of the inferior turbinate bones.

■ THE CONJUNCTIVA (Fig. 5)

The conjunctiva is one continuous thin layer of mucous membrane. It can be divided into three parts:
1 palpebral conjunctiva
2 bulbar conjunctiva
3 fornix.

The palpebral conjunctiva: This consists of two layers – the transparent palpebral layer which contains the lacrimal glands and the epithelial layer.
The bulbar conjunctiva: This covers the anterior part of the eyeball but not the cornea. Here it is very thin and transparent. It does not contain any glands.
The fornix: This is the fold where the palpebral conjunctiva reflects to become the bulbar conjunctiva. It is a loose fold which ensures un-restricted movement of the eyeball. The ducts of the lacrimal gland open into it.

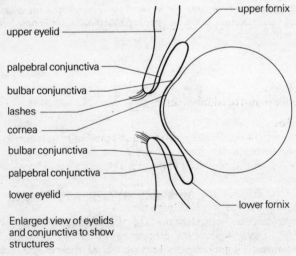

Enlarged view of eyelids and conjunctiva to show structures

Fig. 5 The conjunctiva

- **Blood supply**

There are two main supplies: the posterior conjunctival arteries and the anterior ciliary arteries.

- **Nerve supply**

From the trigeminal (5th cranial) nerve.

■ THE SCLERA (Figs. 1 and 2, p. 4)

The sclera is the tough fibrous outer coat of the eyeball. It is opaque and because of its tough nature gives strength to the globe. At the posterior part of the eyeball, the sclera is pierced by the optic nerve, and the sclera joins with the outer fibrous coat of the nerve. The anterior part of the sclera is covered by the bulbar conjunctiva, and slightly farther back are the insertions of the four rectus muscles and two oblique muscles.

■ PROCEDURES

- **Instillation of drops**

Indications:
   For the administration of drugs for ocular absorption

Requirements:
   Tray or receiver
   Prescribed drops
   Box of tissues
   Notes for record of administration

□ *Procedure*

a Seat the patient comfortably and explain the procedure and the effects of the drops to be given to him.
b Check the patient's identity and the prescription for the drops.
c Wash your hands.
d Ask the patient to tilt his head back and to look upwards; gently pull down the patient's lower lid using a tissue.
e Hold the dropper perpendicular to the patient's eye, a few centimetres away, and gently squeeze the dropper to provide one drop into the lower fornix. (It is important to warn the patient of the insertion of the drop.)
f Ask the patient to close his eye gently.

g Wipe away any excess fluid with a tissue.
h Advise the patient about the effects of the drop, e.g. that mydriatics will cause blurring of vision.

■ Instillation of ointments

Requirements and procedure as for drops but substituting ointment. When instilling ointment start at inner corner and place fine thread of ointment along lower fornix. Warn the patient that the vision will be blurred due to the ointment smearing the cornea.

■ Eye dressing

Indications:
   To promote the patient's comfort.
   To aid healing.
   To protect the eye from injury.

Requirements:
   Clean trolley.
   Sterile eye dressing pack.
   Bottle of Ringer's solution two-thirds strength.
   Sterile eye pad.
   Non-allergic tape to secure the pad.
   Disposal bag.
   Prescribed drops/ointment.
   Torch.
   Patient's notes for recording purposes.

□ *Procedure*
(This is usually carried out in a treatment room, but may be carried out by the patient's bedside.)

a Wash your hands. Tip the dressing pack on to the upper shelf of the trolley; without touching the contents, clip the outer bag on to the side of the trolley to receive soiled dressings.
d Ask the accompanying nurse to pour the Ringer's solution into the relevant receptacle. She should then wash her hands and remove and discard safely the patient's previous dressing. (The lotion must always be checked.)
e Fold the swabs into four, and dip the corner to be used for swabbing into the lotion.
f Ask the patient to look upwards while cleaning his lower eyelid and to look down when cleaning the upper lid margin.

g Swab from the inner to the outer canthus removing any debris on the swabs. All used swabs should be discarded into the disposal bag clipped to the side of the trolley.

h Ask the second nurse to shine the torch to enable examination of the patient's eyes. Examine the anterior segment in a systematic manner and record accurately the findings; changes which have taken place since a previous dressing should be noted.

i If medication has been prescribed this should be checked according to the hospital policy to ensure safe administration.

j Apply an appropriate dressing if necessary.

k Clean the trolley.

l Ensure that the patient is comfortable by evaluation of care at the completion of the procedure.

Note: If an eye pad is to be used always ask the patient to close his eye and to keep it closed while his eye is dressed. Failure to do so may result in a corneal abrasion.

■ Cutting lashes

Indication:

Pre-operatively. This procedure is becoming less commonly used, but some surgeons may request this to be carried out for the patient prior to operation.

Requirements:

Clean trolley.
Drop pack (containing sterile galipot and lint squares).
Ringer's solution.
Tube of sterile soft paraffin.
Eyelash scissors (these have rounded ends).
Patient's nursing notes.

□ *Procedure*

a Explain the procedure to the patient and position him comfortably with his head well supported. Ensure that there is adequate lighting.

b Check the patient's identity and check that the patient has signed his consent form, and that his eye for operation has been marked by the doctor; this is important in order to maintain patient safety, and to fulfil the legal requirements.

c Wash your hands.

d Open the pack and the scissors. Ask the assisting nurse to pour the solution, and place a small amount of the sterile soft paraffin on a swab to wipe the blades of the scissors.

e Ask the patient to look upwards when the lower lashes are being cut; retracting the lid gently cut the lashes, taking care not to traumatize the lid in any way. Wipe the scissors with a swab to remove lashes, put more sterile soft paraffin on to the blades. Ask the patient to look downwards, retract the upper lid gently, and cut the eyelashes from the upper lid margin. Clean the lashes from the scissors using a swab, and discard.

Note: The curved end of the scissors must always be directed away from the eye when cutting the lashes. Lashes should be cut short, but not too close to the lid margin. Sterile soft paraffin is used so that the lashes will adhere to the grease, and not fall into the patient's eye.

f Clean the patient's eyelids, and remove any remaining loose lashes with a moistened swab.

g Examine the patient's eye, using a torch, to ensure that no loose lashes remain.

h Ensure that the patient is comfortable at the end of the procedure.

i Clean away equipment. Wash your hands, and record the procedure in the patient's nursing notes.

■ Conjunctival swab

Indications:
    Pre-operative check.
    To establish the presence of infection

Requirements:
    Sterile conjunctival swab.
    Clean tray.
    Laboratory request slip.
    Relevant medium.

□ *Procedure*

a Explain procedure to patient.

b Label swab with patient's name, date of birth, hospital number and correct eye.

c Remove swab from container, ask patient to look up and run swab lightly along lower fornix.

d Replace in container and send straight to laboratory with the correct form.

e If taking swabs from both eyes, use a second swab and repeat procedure.

In the laboratory, the swab is transferred on to an agar plate and the plate cultured in a warm medium for 24–48 hours until any bacteria can be isolated.

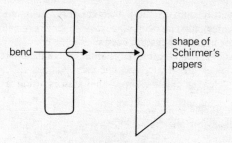

Fig. 6 Schirmer's papers
(Other types of strips may be used)

■ **Schirmer's test**

Indications:
To measure tear secretion for patients with suspected dry eyes.

Requirements:
Sterile Schirmer's strips (Fig. 6).
Scale for reading result.
Tissues.
Sellotape.
Patient's nursing notes.

□ *Procedure*
a Explain the procedure to the patient, and position him with his head well supported.
b Wash your hands.
c Remove the strips from their sterile cover and label the ends 'left' and 'right'. This is to ensure the correct strip is identified for each eye for an accurate assessment of tear secretion.
d Bend the notch of the Schirmer's test strips to a right angle (90°) – this forms a small flap. Ask the patient to look up, and place the flap over the lower lid so that the short piece goes into the lower fornix, the long piece on to the cheek. The patient may continue blinking, but he may find it more comfortable to close his eyes.

Ask the patient not to squeeze his eyes tightly as this may produce a reflex production of tears giving rise to a false reading.
e Leave the Schirmer's test strips in position for 5 minutes, then remove gently and record how far along the paper the moisture has reached. Measure this against the reading scale, and record the result in the

patient's notes as xmm in the 5 minutes (normal is approximately 15mm/5 minutes).

f Stick the strips into the patient's notes.

g Ensure that the patient is comfortable at the end of the procedure.

■ Hot spoon bathing

Indications:
> To reduce inflammation.
> To relieve pain.
> To assist with the absorption of ocular medication.

Requirements:
> Jug of very hot water.
> Large tray.
> Wooden or plastic spoon covered with an eye pad and gauze bandage.
> Tissues.
> Patient's nursing notes.

□ *Procedure*

a Explain this to the patient.

b Supervise the patient, if necessary, to maintain a safe environment and prevent scalding.

c Ask the patient to sit at a table, ensuring that he is comfortable. Place the tray and the jug of very hot water on the table; *ensure that it is secure*, and show the patient how to dip the padded spoon into the water.

d The padded spoon should be held near the patient's affected eye (which should be closed) but should not touch the eyelids as this may result in burning. This action should be repeated at approximately 10-second intervals. The effect of the steam is to dilate the blood vessels, which helps reduce inflammation and thus reduces pain, and assists in the absorption of ocular drugs.

Before the patient leaves the department the nurse must make quite sure that he understands how to continue the treatment at home, 3–4 times daily.

■ Epilation of lashes

Indications:
> To remove eyelashes which are growing inwards (trichiasis) and causing discomfort and damage to the eye.

Requirements:
> Sterile tray.

Tissues.
Sterile epilation forceps.
Magnifier/slit lamp.
Patient's nursing notes.

☐ *Procedure*

a Explain this to the patient, and position him comfortably with his head well supported. Ensure that an adequate light source is available to carry out the procedure.

b Identify the ingrowing lashes with the use of a magnifier or slit lamp.

c Gently hold down the lower lid and ask the patient to look upwards; this is to ensure that no damage is caused to the cornea during the procedure.

d Using the epilation forceps, hold the eyelash close to its base and pull gently forward on the lash to remove it.

e Gently hold the upper lid and ask the patient to look downwards and proceed as for the lower lid.

f Re-examine the patient's lid margins, to ensure that all the ingrowing lashes have been removed.

■ **Eversion of the upper eyelid**

Indications:

This is performed (a) if the patient complains of a foreign body sensation, and (b) during eye irrigation.

Requirements:
Sterile tray.
Tissues.
Glass rod.

☐ *Procedure*

a Explain this to the patient and position him comfortably with his head well supported.

b Wash your hands and stand behind the patient. The patient is told that the procedure may feel a little uncomfortable.

c Hold the lashes of the top eyelid between forefinger and thumb; a glass rod in the other hand is placed on the outer surface of the eyelid and the eyelid turned over the glass rod so that the palpebral conjunctiva can be observed. If this procedure is being carried out during eye irrigation, the inside of the lid should be thoroughly irrigated in order to remove any superficial debris.

d Gently replace the eyelid to its normal position and ask the patient to blink. Ensure he is comfortable afterwards.

■ Rodding

Indications:

To prevent adhesion of the lids to the bulbar conjunctiva (symblepharon). This occurs as a complication of chemical and heat burns.

Requirements:

Sterile tray.
Sterile glass rods.
Lubricant, e.g. soft paraffin or other prescribed ointment.
Local anaesthetic eyedrops, e.g. amethocaine 1%.
Patient's nursing notes.

□ *Procedure*

a Explain this to the patient, emphasize the importance of continuing regular daily treatment. Position the patient comfortably with his head well supported.

b Wash your hands and instil the prescribed, and checked, local anaesthetic eyedrop to anaesthetize the patient's eye prior to rodding.

c Lubricate the lip of the glass rod and ask the patient to look upwards while the glass rod is gently inserted into the lower fornix.

d Using a gentle sweeping movement, move the glass rod several times along the length of the lower eyelid. If requested by the doctor, repeat this procedure in the patient's upper fornix.

e Apply prescribed ointment generously to maintain lubrication between the palpebral and bulbar conjunctiva.

f Ensure that the patient is comfortable, and that he understands the importance of follow-up care and continuity of treatment.

■ Eye irrigation

Indications:

To irrigate the patient's eye following chemical burns.
To remove foreign materials from the eye.
To cool the eye after heat burns.

Requirements:

Clean trolley.
Sterile dressing pack.
Protective cape for the patient.
Sterile Fischer's dish.
Plastic undine.
Appropriate solution at room temperature, e.g. universal buffer solution.
Local anaesthetic eyedrops, e.g. amethocaine 1%.

Universal indicator tape.
Gauze swabs.
Dressed orange sticks.
Patient's nursing notes.

In hospital the procedure is carried out using the sterile equipment listed. Because rapid action is required at the time of an accident clean tap water may be used so as not to delay irrigation.

This is an emergency situation as chemical substances and other foreign material may endanger the patient's sight.

□ *Procedure*

a Explain this promptly to the patient while starting treatment.

b Position him comfortably with his head well supported. If he is in a great deal of pain, a local anaesthetic drop is instilled into his eye.

c Quickly cover the patient's clothing with a protective cape.

d Check the tear pH with an indicator strip, and enter this in the patient's notes. This is to assess acidity/alkalinity of tears prior to irrigation.

e Prepare the dressing pad. Fill the undine with the appropriate solution.

f The Fischer's dish should be held next to the patient's cheek to receive the solution during irrigation. The patient should be asked to turn his head to the affected side.

g Test the solution first on the patient's cheek so that he can feel the temperature of the fluid before it is run into his eye.

h Hold the lower eyelid down gently. Ask the patient to look in all directions while irrigating his eye. The upper eyelid should be everted to irrigate the inside surface.

i Any solid particles should be removed gently with the dressed orange stick.

j Swab the eyelids after irrigation.

k Re-check the tear pH and record this in the patient's notes. (Irrigation should be repeated if the tear pH has not returned to normal.)

l After completion of the procedure the patient's visual acuity should be checked.

■ Syringing of the lacrimal sac

Indications:

To assess the patency of the nasolacrimal passages.

To flush out mucopurulent matter where the patient has chronic inflammation of the nasolacrimal passages (dacryocystitis).

To introduce antibiotics for the treatment of dacryocystitis.

For radiological purposes, e.g. dacryocystogram.

Requirements:
    Clean trolley.
    Sterile dressing pack.
    2ml syringe.
    Lacrimal syringing set which contains:
        1 Nettleship dilator;
        2 lacrimal cannula.
    Ringer's solution.
    Prescribed drugs, e.g. antibiotics.
    Prescribed local anaesthetic eyedrops, e.g. amethocaine 1%.
    Patient's nursing notes.

□ *Procedure*
a Explain this to the patient and help him into a comfortable position with his head well supported and tilted slightly backwards.
b Wash your hands, and instil prescribed local anaesthetic drops directly over the punctum to be syringed.
c Position the towel to protect the patient's clothing.
d Ask the patient to look upwards during the procedure, to protect the cornea.
e Insert the Nettleship dilator into the patient's lower punctum and follow the passage of the canaliculus rotating the dilator gently during this process. Withdraw the dilator when the punctum is dilated.
    Note: Warn the patient that during introduction of the solution he may experience a salty taste.
f Insert the lacrimal cannula in the same way as the Nettleship dilator; inject the solution very gently.
g As the solution is inserted ask the patient whether he can feel water at the back of his throat. If so, tell him to swallow it. If it is not possible to pass any fluid along the lacrimal canal the patient should be referred back to the doctor.
    Note: From the ability or otherwise of the water to flow it is possible to determine that:
        i If the patient swallows water the duct is patent.
        ii If the patient does not feel water in his throat, or the water regurgitates through the upper punctum, then the duct is blocked.
        iii It is not possible to syringe the duct at all.
h Record carefully all results. If both lacrimal passages are being syringed, a separate cannula should be used for each to avoid the possible transmission of infection.

■ Sub-conjunctival injection

Indications:

> To facilitate rapid absorption of ocular drugs allowing them to enter the aqueous fluid in higher concentrations than if administered in the form of eyedrops.
>
> It is useful in the treatment of acute inflammatory disorders of the eye. Injection of prophylactic antibiotics may also be administered by this route.
>
> Following some surgical procedures according to the wishes of the individual surgeon.
>
> To maintain pupil dilation (mydriasis).

Requirements:

> Clean trolley or tray.
> Sterile dressing pad.
> 2ml syringe.
> No 21g needle for drawing up the solution for injection.
> No 25g needle for injection of the prescribed medication.
> Paraffin gauze.
> Eye pad.
> Tape.
> Bandage (if required).
> Prescribed medication.
> Patient's prescription chart and nursing notes.

□ *Procedure*

a Explain this to the patient. It should be remembered that the anticipation of this treatment may be very frightening for the patient so the nurse must deal with this in a very sensitive and gently efficient manner.

b Position the patient comfortably with his head well supported.

c Wash your hands and instil the prescribed local anaesthetic drops.

d Draw up the prescribed, and checked, drug for injection, and change to a 25g needle.

e Direct the needle horizontally, with the bevel of the needle uppermost, and insert into the subconjunctival space. The bevel should remain in view, but should be covered by the transparent conjunctiva. Inject the drug gently, having previously indicated to the patient that he may experience a sensation of pressure, which is the result of the ballooning of the conjunctiva during the instillation of the injection fluid.

f Apply paraffin gauze and an eye pad, ensuring that the patient's eye is closed underneath the pad. Advise the patient to remove the pad after four hours if necessary. (A bandage will sometimes also be required following this procedure.)

■ **Retrobulbar injection**

This procedure is *always* carried out by a medical practitioner.

Indications:
>   To relieve a blind painful eye when the patient does not wish to have the eye removed. This is not a procedure to be undertaken lightly and the decision to perform it will have resulted from the doctor's and patient's discussion.
>
>   Prior to surgery under local anaesthetic.
>
>   Local anaesthetic in theatre before photocoagulation.

Requirements:
>   Trolley or tray.
>   Hibitane in spirit.
>   Sterile dressing pack.
>   Syringes and needles.
>   Retrobulbar needle.
>   Medication for injection.
>   Local anaesthetic.
>   Savlon for skin preparation.

□ *Procedure*
a Explain this to the patient.
b Clean trolley and lay up.
c The doctor washes his hands and dries them on the sterile towel. The skin area of injection is prepared and the second sterile towel is placed on the patient.
d The skin is anaesthetized locally using 2% lignocaine with adrenaline prior to the retrobulbar injection's being given.
e The doctor gives the injection in the region of the ciliary ganglion and muscle cone. If given for absolute glaucoma 70% or 90% alcohol is used. If given as a local anaesthetic before surgery, lignocaine hydrochloride 2% and adrenaline is used.
f If performed in the outpatient department make sure the patient is well before he goes home and preferably has an escort.

■ **PRACTICE QUESTIONS**

1 *Are the following true or false?*
>   a Eyelids are made up of layers.
>   b Eyelids contain glands.
>   c Sweat glands are known as Zeis.

    d The eyelids have no function.
    e Tears are secreted from the conjunctiva.
    f Tears keep the cornea moist.
    g The lacrimal glands are situated in a depression in the frontal bone.
    h The glands are about the size of an almond.
    i There are 20 ducts which conduct tears.
    j Tears are just made up of water.
    k There is one punctum in each eyelid.
    l The conjunctiva is one continuous thin layer of mucous membrane.
    m The conjunctiva can be divided into three parts.
    n The nerve supply to the conjunctiva is the 4th cranial nerve.
    o The sclera is the innermost layer of the eye.
    p The sclera is opaque.
    q The anterior part of the sclera is covered by the bulbar conjunctiva.
    r Eyelashes are attached to the lid margins.
    s Blinking washes away any dust which may be in the conjunctival sac.

2 *Answer the following questions*

    a Name the layers that comprise the eyelid.
    b Name the two types of gland the eyelids contain.
    c What are the functions of the eyelids?
    d What is the function of the lacrimal apparatus?
    e Where does the nasolacrimal duct open?
    f Name the three parts of the conjunctiva.
    g Which part of the conjunctiva contains the lacrimal glands and on to which part do they open?
    h Describe the sclera.
    i What nerve pierces the sclera on the posterior segment of the eye?
    j What muscles have their insertions on the sclera?
    k List requirements for the instillation of eyedrops.
    l When instilling ointment at which corner of the eye do you start?
    m List requirements for laying up a basic eye dressing trolley.
    n What is very important before putting an eye pad on?
    o List requirements for cutting lashes.
    p Why would you take conjunctival swabs?
    q How would you take conjunctival swabs?
    r For what reason is a Schirmer's test performed? List what items are needed.
    s Name a method of heat application.
    t Why would you epilate lashes?
    u Describe how you would evert the upper eyelid.
    v Why is an eye irrigated?
    w For what reason would you perform a lacrimal sac washout?

  x After a lacrimal sac washout what three reasons would lead you to suspect the nasolacrimal duct is blocked?

  y What do you understand by the term sub-conjunctival injection?

  z For what reasons would a sub-conjunctival injection be given?

 aa What do you understand by the term 'retrobulbar' injection? Which member of staff would give this injection?

 bb For what reasons is a retrobulbar injection given?

■ **Answers**

1 *a* True   *f* True   *k* True   *p* True
  b True   *g* True   *l* True   *q* True
  c False   *h* True   *m* True   *r* True
  d False   *i* False   *n* False   *s* True
  e True   *j* False   *o* False

2 *a* Skin, loose connective tissue, muscle, tarsal plate, fascia and palpebral conjunctiva.

  b Sebaceous, called Zeis. Sweat, called Moll.

  c (i) protective; (ii) lubrication; (iii) cleansing.

  d To drain away the tears.

  e Into the nasal cavity.

  f Palpebral, bulbar and the fornix.

  g The palpebral conjunctiva contains the lacrimal glands and they open into the fornix.

  h The sclera is the tough fibrous outer coat of the eyeball.

  i The optic nerve.

  j The four rectus muscles and two oblique muscles.

  k Sterile cardboard tray or receiver, cotton-wool balls, correct eye-drops.

  l Start at inner corner and squeeze a fine line of ointment to outer corner.

  m Trolley and tray. Hibitane 1 : 2000 in 70% spirit for cleaning trolley, sterile eye pack, saline, non-allergic tape, crêpe or gauze bandage (if needed), correct drops/ointment, torch, prescription chart.

  n Asking the patient to close his eye, to avoid risk of a corneal abrasion.

  o Sterile cardboard tray or receiver, pair round-ended scissors, tube of soft paraffin, pack of gauze swabs.

  p For sticky eyes, and as a routine pre-operative check.

  q Explain procedure to patient, label swab with patient's name, date of birth, hospital number and correct eye. Remove swab from container, ask patient to look up and run swab lightly along the lower fornix. Replace in container, send straight to laboratory with correct form. If taking swabs from both eyes, use a second swab and repeat procedure.

r A Schirmer's test is recorded if a patient complains of dry irritable eyes and the doctor suspects that the lacrimal gland is not working properly. Items needed are: pack of Schirmer's papers and a paper measure.

s Hot spoon bathing.

t To remove lashes that are causing discomfort and damage to the patient's eye.

u Make patient comfortable, and the nurse stands behind the patient. Explain what you are going to do. The lashes are held between the forefinger and thumb, a glass rod in the other hand is placed on the outer surface of the eyelid and the eyelid turned over the glass rod so that the palpebral conjunctiva can be seen. To return the eyelid to normal, it is just brushed gently and the patient is told to blink.

v To remove any foreign materials causing further damage to the eye.

w It is suspected that the patient has blocked tear ducts and the patient complains of watering eyes.

x *i* Patient does not feel water in throat.
  ii Water regurgitates in upper punctum.
  iii Unable to syringe at all.

y An injection given through the conjunctiva so that the fluid lies between the conjunctiva and the sclera.

z Hypopyon; to dilate a stubborn pupil; synechia; to reduce inflammation; at time of surgery.

aa Retrobulbar injection is given into the region of the ciliary ganglion and muscle cone behind the eye.
  It is given by a member of the medical staff.

bb To relieve a blind painful eye; prior to surgery under local anaesthetic; as a local anaesthetic in theatre before photocoagulation.

3 Outpatients, accident and emergency care and minor operative procedures

■ RECEPTION OF PATIENTS IN THE OPHTHALMIC DEPARTMENT

As a result of changes which have occurred in recent years in ophthalmic medical and surgical practice, as well as advances in technology, the emphasis of patient care is in many cases being redirected towards outpatient treatment. This will obviously have profound effects on nurses' attitudes to their roles in the ophthalmic department.

These changes call for individual care, in-depth nursing assessment, patient education, and evaluation to meet the needs of outpatients.

People coming to the ophthalmic department for the first time may be rather apprehensive, especially if their sight has deteriorated rapidly prior to their appointment. It is, therefore, very important that the approach of the nurse is both gently efficient and sensitive, with emphasis on effective communication.

Ocular trauma represents an important area in ophthalmic nursing care, and the extent of this problem is often underestimated. It should be remembered that where ocular trauma has taken place the patient may experience considerable pain and may be very distressed and fearful. Other injuries may also be present and, importantly, neurological complications may be associated with ocular trauma.

Nursing assessment plays a very important part in both the outpatient and the accident and emergency departments. Immediate assessment of the problem in the latter is vital if essential priorities of care are to be achieved. The implementation of a triage system in some departments has greatly facilitated this. It must be remembered that ocular trauma, if associated with other injuries, may be life-threatening while other ocular emergencies will be sight-threatening. Nursing assessment, must take account of the person, his individual needs, his understanding of his condition, and his social setting, within which he may be required to continue treatment.

Before seeing the doctor, the following observations may be recorded:
1 Visual acuity.

2 Blood pressure.

3 Urinalysis.

The recording of the person's visual acuity should always be carried out as soon as possible, and before medical examination and treatment take place. The exception to this is where the patient requires immediate eye irrigation, after which the patient's visual acuity must be assessed and recorded. Accurate recording of visual acuity is essential to provide a basis against which comparison may be made at a later stage of care and should be carried out for medico-legal purposes.

Initial ocular examination is carried out and recorded. This is often initiated by the nurse prior to medical examination, and completed in detail by the doctor. Experienced ophthalmic nurses will be able to use the slit lamp for this purpose. In any case, an adequate light source to aid eye examination is important.

Examination of the patient's eyes should always be carried out in a systematic manner, observing:

Lids.

Conjunctiva.

Cornea.

Iris/anterior chamber.

Pupils (size, shape and reaction to light).

Lens ⎫ detailed examination of these structures

Vitreous ⎬ requires observation by the doctor using

Retina ⎭ the slit lamp and ophthalmoscope.

Wherever possible the nurse should accompany the patient to explain any examination and treatment to be carried out and to ensure his comfort.

Following medical examination, treatment may be required. Very often ophthalmic treatment will require the patient to continue care at home; in this case it is essential that the nurse assesses the patient's ability to do so, since compliance with continuing treatment will be vital to the patient's recovery, and to the prevention of complications. Teaching and supervision should be based on the nursing assessment, and its effectiveness evaluated to ensure that the patient's needs have been met.

■ OPHTHALMIC TRAUMA AND ACUTE CONDITIONS

■ Corneal abrasion

The patient presents with a pink, watering eye. Visual acuity is recorded and the patient examined on the slit lamp. The eye is examined, local

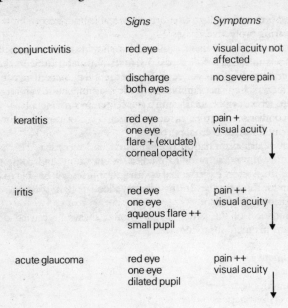

	Signs	Symptoms
conjunctivitis	red eye	visual acuity not affected
	discharge both eyes	no severe pain
keratitis	red eye one eye flare + (exudate) corneal opacity	pain + visual acuity
iritis	red eye one eye aqueous flare ++ small pupil	pain ++ visual acuity
acute glaucoma	red eye one eye dilated pupil	pain ++ visual acuity

Fig. 7 Causes of red eye

anaesthetic drops are instilled and fluorescein staining carried out. This will show up green if there is an abrasion.

□ *Treatment*

Mydriatic drops, e.g. homatropine 1%, and antibiotic drops, e.g. chloramphenicol (Chloromycetin) to the affected eye. Pad and bandage are supplied. A letter for the GP will be written and drops given to take home. Removal of the pad is at the doctor's discretion, depending on the severity of the abrasion. Instructions are given to the patient on instillation of drops. He may or may not be seen again in the clinic.

■ **Foreign body**

□ *Corneal*

A nursing assessment should be carried out and the patient's history is recorded; the visual acuity in both eyes is assessed. This is important as often patients make industrial claims if the injury happened at work and sometimes the case will go to court. Also establish and record if the patient was wearing protective glasses.

The patient is examined by the doctor and seated by the slit lamp. Amethocaine 1% is instilled and a fluorescein strip placed in the lower fornix and removed. (Some departments use 1% fluorescein eyedrops.)

The patient's eye is examined with the slit lamp and the foreign body removed (if it is embedded using a hypodermic needle gauge 17). If the foreign body is steel or metal a rust ring should be looked for and removed.

After removal of the object chloramphenicol (eyedrops or ointment) and a mydriatic drop, e.g. homatropine 1% or Mydrilate 1% (to relieve ciliary muscle spasm) are instilled and a pad applied firmly. The patient is advised when to remove the pad and a prescription given for either drops or ointment, and a letter for the GP. Depending on the damage to the eye from the foreign body, the doctor will decide whether he wishes to see the patient again.

□ *Conjunctival*

The patient presents complaining of:

   i 'Something in the eye'.

  ii Watering eye.

 iii Pink eye.

On examination the foreign body may be seen in the lower or upper fornix after eversion of the lid. After instillation of amethocaine 1% eyedrops it can be removed with a cotton bud. If it is not seen the upper eyelid is everted and checked. A corneal foreign body should be excluded.

If the patient still complains of irritation, the eye can be irrigated using saline and chloramphenicol ointment instilled.

■ **Stye (external hordeolum)**

This is a staphylococcal infection in the gland of Zeis. The patient presents with a red painful swelling of upper and lower lid. Visual acuity is recorded and the patient advised to carry out hot spoon bathing and chloramphenicol ointment three times a day is prescribed. If the patient complains of recurrent styes, his urine should be tested for glucose and ketones, as diabetics often develop this condition and the patient may be an unknown diabetic.

■ **Conjunctivitis** (Fig. 7)

Often a patient is referred to an ophthalmic department with this condition. The patient presents with an uncomfortable eye with a 'gritty' sensation; the eye(s) may be red and watering profusely; either one or both eyes may be affected.

□ *Nursing and medical care*

The visual acuity is assessed and the result recorded accurately. Any foreign body should be excluded.

Chloramphenicol eyedrops/ointment is prescribed for the affected eye(s). If drops for both eyes are prescribed two bottles should be dispensed labelled left and right.

A further outpatient appointment is not necessary unless the condition persists.

This condition is very contagious and the patient should be advised to keep anything personal away from the remainder of the family, e.g. towels and flannels, and is advised not to wear make-up.

■ **Iritis** (Fig. 7)

This is inflammation of the iris. The patient presents with a red, painful, watering eye; the pupil is usually miosed.

The visual acuity is diminished.

The visual acuity is recorded and the patient examined by the doctor. The patient is then examined on the slit lamp and the finding recorded.

□ *Treatment*

The pupil is dilated using mydriatic drops, e.g. homatropine 1% or Mydrilate 1%; chloramphenicol and Predsol are also instilled. If the iritis is severe a sub-conjunctival injection may be given. The patient will be more comfortable if the eye is padded. The patient is treated as an out-patient if the condition is not too severe. But if the patient is very uncomfortable with a severe iritis it is best to admit him, continue the treatment described above and apply local heat.

Analgesics may also be required initially.

The patient is discharged when the iritis has subsided.

■ **Arc eye**

This occurs as a result of welding usually where protective goggles have not been worn. A sudden flash of light is directed into the face. Both eyes are usually affected. Patients present with pink, watering eyes, and feel very uncomfortable.

□ *Treatment*

The visual acuity is recorded, and the patient is examined by the doctor. Chloramphenicol or an alternative antibiotic ointment is prescribed.

■ Corneal ulcer

These are caused by:

a Bacteria, e.g. *Diplococcus pneumoniae* (pneumococcus); *Betahaemolytic streptococcus*; *Bacillus pyocyaneus*; *Moraxella liquefaciens*; *Klebsiella pneumoniae*.

b Viruses, e.g. herpes simplex (dendritic ulcer); vaccinia (rare).

c Fungi, e.g. *Candida albicans* (monilia); aspergillus; cephalosporium.

d Hypersensitivity reactions, e.g. to staphylococci (marginal ulcer); to unknown allergens or toxins; to tubercular protein and, rarely, other bacterial proteins (phlyctenular-kerato conjunctivitis).

e Vitamin deficiency, e.g. (avitaminosis A (xerophthalmia)).

f Nerve lesions, e.g. of the 5th cranial (neurotrophic).

g Exposure.

h Unknown causes such as Moorens ulcer.

Generally the patient presents with any or all of these signs and symptoms:

Redness

Pain

Photophobia

Excessive lacrimation

Diminished visual acuity.

The eye is examined and the ulcer identified by means of fluorescein staining.

□ *Treatment*

This can be as an inpatient or as an outpatient. A pad or dark glasses depending on the severity of the ulcer should be worn. Drops and/or ointment. Mydriatics, e.g. Mydrilate or homatropine 1% to dilate the pupil and prevent iritis and posterior synechia (adhesion of iris to lens).

Antibiotics, e.g. chloramphenicol.

Anti-viral, e.g. idoxuridine, Vira-A.

Steroids, e.g. Predsol/Betnesol.

Analgesia as required.

The frequency of medication will depend on the doctor's instruction.

If the ulcer does not respond to drop treatment, sub-conjunctival injection may be indicated (see p. 29).

In the case of some viral ulcers, debridement of the ulcer may be necessary.

■ Burns

This is one incident where the patient's visual acuity is not recorded until immediate treatment has been carried out. The source of the burns should be ascertained whether acid or alkali. The patient is seated or lain on a couch if shocked; amethocaine 1% eyedrops are instilled to relieve the pain and immediate irrigation commenced using saline or buffer solution, or sodium versonate 0.4% to dissolve lime. If it is an acid burn the acid will be washed out fairly quickly; if it is an alkali burn, e.g. lime, the eye must be irrigated for at least 15 to 20 minutes as lime deposits continue to burn and may cause deep corneal damage.

When the doctor is satisfied that the irrigation is sufficient, visual acuity is recorded, the patient's eye examined and chloramphenicol ointment instilled and the eye padded. The patient will probably require analgesia such as Panadol, and admission is advised.

The patient is seen daily by the doctor and rodding (to reduce symblepharon) two–three times a day may be requested. While an inpatient the patient may be up and about and eventually the eye pad replaced by dark glasses.

The patient will be asked to return to the department for a check-up.

■ Penetrating/perforating injuries

□ *Assessment*

The patient will come to the department after an injury to his eye. The eye appears to water – this may not be tears but aqueous escaping from the anterior chamber. Sometimes the eye settles down and the patient does not come to the department for a few days, so it is important to establish when and where the injury happened, and to record it, also to establish whether the patient was wearing spectacles or protective glasses.

Visual acuity is recorded and the patient carefully examined by the doctor and as accurate a history obtained as possible. No pressure should be put on the eye at any time. The following details should be recorded:

1 Visual acuity.
2 Date when accident happened.
3 Approximate time of injury.
4 Any protection worn?
5 Type of material used and action taken, e.g. hammering, welding.

□ *Aids to diagnosis*

1 The patient is moved as little as possible.
2 Examination by ophthalmoscope.
3 Examination by slit lamp.
4 Radiological examination of eye and orbit.

□ *Diagnosis*

1 Decide whether entry of foreign body was via cornea or sclera.

2 Locate wound – corneal wounds will be seen, scleral wounds not always.
3 Check the radiograph to see if the foreign body is radio-opaque and define area where the foreign body is lodged.

□ *Admission*
1 Advise the patient as to the diagnosis, treatment and prognosis. Arrange immediate admission and ask the doctor to explain any procedures and sign the consent form with the patient. Contact the patient's relatives. Admit the patient and carry out a full nursing assessment.
2 A course of systemic antibiotics is commenced. Surgery will be necessary at an early time but need not be immediate. Care should be taken when moving the patient.

□ *Theatre*
The patient is anaesthetized and placed on the operating table. The lashes will be cut if the surgeon wishes. The eye is prepared and the surgeon removes the foreign body using the technique which he thinks is most appropriate. If the foreign body is magnetic it will be possible to withdraw it using a hand magnet or the larger DC (direct current) magnet. If it is non-magnetic, its position will decide whether it is possible to remove it. Vitrectomy may be performed.

□ *Postoperative*
The patient is returned to his bed, made comfortable and general post-operative care carried out, e.g.
  observations of pulse, blood pressure and respirations;
  check for vomiting;
  observe dressing but do not remove.
The doctor will have written up the operation notes and these and any postoperative instructions regarding movement of the patient should be followed.

The first dressing is usually performed about 24 hours from the time of surgery. The patient is kept comfortable in the position that has been ordered, which may be lying down or sitting up. His toilet requirements are attended to; it is better to give regular gentle face wipes. Offer a bed pan/urinal; washing of hands, and care of pressure areas rather than an extensive bed bath until the condition of the eye has been seen. Teeth brushing is inadvisable, gentle mouthwashing every couple of hours is preferable.

Early mobilization is used and will be indicated by the surgeon.

Earphones are provided for the radio. When approaching the patient ensure that he is aware of your presence. Do *not* take him by surprise!

□ *First dressing*

The trolley is prepared as for the basic eye dressing (p. 20), and in addition a pair of stitch scissors and suture forceps are placed on the base of the trolley, and the trolley taken to the bedside.

Explain the procedure to the patient, slide inner eye pack on to the top of the trolley and fix outer bag for soiled dressings. Ask a second nurse to remove the patient's dressing while hands are washed and dried on sterile towel from pack. Place second towel on patient.

The dressing should be inspected before being discarded; the patient will probably have his eyelids covered with a piece of tulle gras (paraffin gauze) which should be removed with the forceps. The lids may have lid sutures (Fig. 8) in place to prevent the patient from opening his eye under the pad.

The same principle applies when removing lid sutures as to any other part of the body, i.e. suture cut next to skin and pulled through.

The eyelids are cleansed gently and the patient warned that his eye will water when opened.

The assistant is asked to shine the torch – first on the cheek and then upwards to the eye. The eye will be red and the tissues chemosed (swollen). The nurse should note the condition of all structures of the anterior part of the eye and check the wound to ensure there is no prolapse of tissue. Check also for hyphaema (blood in anterior chamber).

Ask the patient if he can see the light.

The drops or ointment prescribed, e.g. Genticin, are instilled and the tulle gras replaced, then an eye pad, tape, bandage or Cartella shield. (These are plastic shields designed to protect the eye.)

Very often the doctor will be present at this dressing to check the condition of the eye to reduce the amount of times the eye is disturbed. If

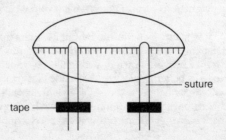

Fig. 8 Lid sutures

all is satisfactory the patient may start to mobilize gradually. Each injury is different and the surgical technique for removal, so there is no hard and fast rule for ambulation.

Eyedrops used will be mydriatics, steroids or antibiotics. The full course of systemic antibiotics is given. The patient is discharged when the doctor is satisfied that the eye has settled down and will be followed-up carefully. He is usually given antibiotic, steroid and mydriatic drops to continue using at home. Dark glasses may be worn. Advice will be given not to bend, stoop or strain.

□ *Complications*
1 Hyphaema (blood in anterior chamber).
2 Vitreous haemorrhage.
3 Hypopyon (pus in anterior chamber).
4 Acute glaucoma.
5 Damage to lens – traumatic cataract.
6 *Phthisis bulbi* (eye collapses and becomes shrunken).
7 Sympathetic ophthalmia (the 'good' eye shows a similar inflammation to the one which has sustained the perforated injury). The injured eye is removed.

■ Diabetes and ocular complications

As all nurses will know, some diabetic patients present with a number of secondary complications. Below is a list of the more common ocular signs connected with diabetes:
Recurrent styes and boils.
Sub-conjunctival haemorrhages.
Iritis.
Iridocyclitis.
Glaucoma.
Cataracts.
Choroiditis.
Vitreous haemorrhage.
Detachments of the retina.
Optic neuritis.
Retinopathy.

■ Ophthalmia neonatorum

This occurs in newborn babies and presents as a purulent conjunctivitis. It is a notifiable disease.

□ *Cause and treatment*

Infection from the mother's genital tract during birth.
Infection following birth during the first three weeks.
Gonococcus/staphylococcus/viral infection.

The baby is seen to have bilateral sticky eyes within a few days of birth. Conjunctival swabs will be taken from both eyes and treatment commenced immediately. Penicillin 1000–2500 IU/ml instilled into both eyes; in the beginning the drops may be instilled as often as two-hourly and then reduced as the condition improves. If both eyes are being treated it is important to have two bottles of drops, one for each eye to prevent any further cross-infection.

■ MINOR OPERATIVE PROCEDURES

■ Tarsorrhaphy

This is the stitching together of the eyelids to protect the cornea. It may be:
a lateral
b central
c medial.

It is performed for:
a corneal ulcer
b dry eye
c anaesthetic cornea – (due to damage of the ophthalmic branch of the trigeminal nerve (5th cranial)).

The patient's lids are sutured together under local anaesthetic, and the sutures removed in the outpatient department 5 to 7 days later. The tarsorrhaphy may be temporary or permanent.

■ Incision and curettage of meibomian cyst

This is a swelling of a meibomian gland following obstruction of its duct accompanied by chronic inflammation of surrounding tissues.

The patient presents with a painless swelling in his eyelid which is adherent to the tarsal plate.

The cyst is removed under local anaesthetic, the eye covered with a pad until the patient gets home and chloramphenicol ointment is instilled twice a day for two days.

■ Electrolysis

This is to remove ingrowing eyelashes. It is done under local anaesthetic using an electrolysis machine.

■ **Cautery**

This is performed using a hand cautery for removal of warts and papilloma and the eversion of punctum. It is performed under a local anaesthetic.

■ **Entropion**

This is where the upper or lower lid turns in, causing the patient problems with lashes, blinking, general discomfort, and carries a risk of corneal abrasion. Under local anaesthetic a cautery or a corrective operation to remove skin and muscle is performed. The skin sutures are removed after 5 days and the patient reviewed.

■ **Ectropion**

This is where the upper or lower lid turns out. The patient is unable to close the eye properly. It causes corneal exposure. Under local anaesthetic cautery or a corrective operation is performed. The sutures are removed according to the individual patient's requirements.

■ **Probing**

This is counted as a minor operation but performed under general anaesthetic. It is done to relieve blocked nasolacrimal ducts where lacrimal syringing has revealed a blockage. The blockage will be passed down the nasolacrimal duct. A series of double-ended probes with different size ends are passed down through the punctum until the obstruction is met and then that probe used to dislodge the obstruction. The patient is usually discharged in the evening or next day.

■ **Ptosis**

The patient presents with drooping of an upper eyelid. He is able to close his eye but has difficulty in opening it fully.

Causes:
1 Congenital.
2 Myasthenia gravis.
3 Increase in the weight of the eyelid, e.g. cyst.
4 Paralysis of the levator muscle.
Corrective oculo-plastic surgery will be necessary except in the case of myasthenia gravis. If the latter is suspected, 1ml Prostigmin is injected. If the ptosis improves or disappears but recurs later, the diagnosis is confirmed.

■ **Biopsy**

This minor surgical procedure is performed under local anaesthetic. Biopsies are taken for warts, suspected rodent ulcers and anything which the doctor wants checked. The specimen is placed in normal saline, labelled and sent to the laboratory with the appropriate form and the patient given a follow-up appointment for the result.

■ PRACTICE QUESTIONS

1 Name three investigations that a new patient may require in the outpatient department.
2 What structures are observed on an objective examination of the eye?
3 A patient presents with a pink, watering eye. The doctor states this is a corneal abrasion. How do you establish that it is an abrasion and how will it be treated?
4 If a patient presents complaining of a foreign body, what is an important fact that should be established?
5 In which of the following four conditions is the visual acuity not affected?
   a conjunctivitis
   b keratitis
   c iritis
   d acute glaucoma.
6 The following are secondary complications of what disease?
   a recurrent styes and boils
   b cataracts
   c retinal detachments
   d retinopathy.
7 If a patient presented with a history of recurrent styes what might you suspect and what simple test could you do?
8 If a foreign body is steel or metal what should you check for?
9 What is a stye and what heat method would you recommend to the patient?
10 What would a patient with conjunctivitis complain of, and what treatment is instituted? What would you advise your patient to do at home?
11 What is iritis? What does the patient present with?
12 What treatment is recommended for a patient with iritis?
13 Give the signs and symptoms of a patient with a corneal ulcer.
14 What staining agent would show a corneal ulcer?
15 Which will burn longer, acid or alkali?

16 In a burns case would you record the visual acuity straight away?

17 What solutions can you use to irrigate an eye?

18 If the burn is thought to be from lime, how long would you irrigate?

19 What complication could happen as a result of the burn and what method would you use to reduce it?

20 A patient may come to the department with a history of an injury and complain that his eye is watering. It may not be tears. What else might it be?

21 What investigations will be carried out if an intra-ocular foreign body is suspected?

22 Name the two types of magnet that may be used to remove the foreign body.

23 What is a tarsorrhaphy? Give the three areas where it may be sutured. When is it done?

24 Describe the difference between an entropion and an ectropion.

25 What is a meibomian cyst? What is the term for removal of this cyst?

26 Would a probing be performed under general or local anaesthetic?

27 What do you understand by the word ptosis, what are the causes?

28 If myasthenia gravis is suspected what injection can be given to confirm the diagnosis?

29 A patient attends the accident and emergency department with a history of 'an injury to the eye'. After initial examination it is thought to be a perforating injury:

   a What investigations will be performed immediately?

   b How is the diagnosis made?

   c Describe this patient's care from admission.

30 What do you understand by:

   a photophobia

   b excessive lacrimation

   c synechia?

■ **Answers**

1 Visual acuity with and without distance glasses. Blood pressure and urinalysis.

2 Lids, conjunctiva, cornea, iris/anterior chamber, lens, retina.

3 The eye is examined, local anaesthetic is instilled and fluorescein staining done. The patient is examined on the slit lamp and the abrasion will show up green. Treatment consists of mydriatics, and antibiotic drops, e.g. homatropine 1% and chloramphenicol. Pad and bandage are provided. Treatment should continue at home and removal of pad and bandage is at the patient's own discretion. A letter

for the GP is provided. The patient is instructed on how to instil drops.

4 Whether the patient was wearing protective glasses and if the injury happened at work.

5 *a*

6 Diabetes.

7 Patient might be diabetic and urinalysis may indicate this.

8 Rust ring.

9 A stye is a staphylococcal infection in the gland of Zeis. Hot spoon bathing would be recommended 2–3 times daily.

10 Patient with conjunctivitis complains of an uncomfortable gritty feeling in both eyes. Red eye, watering profusely.
   Treatment: Check visual acuity. Exclude foreign body and prescribe chloramphenicol eyedrops or ointment.
   At home: Condition is contagious so patient should keep flannels, towels, etc, away from other members of the family. Advised not to wear make-up.

11 Iritis is inflammation of the iris. The patient presents with a red, painful, watering eye, the pupil is miosed and the visual acuity diminished.

12 Dilate pupil with mydriatic eyedrops, e.g. Mydrilate 1% or homatropine 1%; give antibiotic eyedrops, e.g. chloramphenicol, and steroid eyedrops, e.g. Predsol. If a severe attack, a sub-conjunctival injection will be given. Pad the eye. Treat as an outpatient if not severe. If a severe attack, admit, continue treatment and apply local heat to give relief. Give analgesics. Discharge when iritis subsided.

13 Redness, pain, photophobia, excessive lacrimation, diminished visual acuity.

14 Fluorescein.

15 Alkali.

16 No, irrigate eye first.

17 Tap water if nothing else available or saline. Buffer solution. If a lime burn use sodium versonate 0.4% to dissolve the lime.

18 At least 15–20 minutes and carry on longer if not satisfied.

19 Complication of burn would be symblepharon. Method used to reduce it would be rodding.

20 Aqueous humour.

21 The patient is moved as little as possible.
   Examination by ophthalmoscope.
   Examination by slit lamp.
   Radiological examination of eye and orbit.

22 Hand magnet and the larger direct current magnet.

23 A tarsorrhaphy is the stitching together of the eyelids to protect the cornea. It may be lateral, central or medial. It is done for corneal ulcer, dry eye, anaesthetic cornea.

24 Entropion is where the upper or lower lid turns in. Ectropion is where the upper or lower lid turns out.

25 A meibomian cyst is a swelling of a meibomian gland following obstruction of its duct accompanied by chronic inflammation of the surrounding tissues. The correct name for removal is incision and curettage.

26 General anaesthetic.

27 Ptosis means drooping of an eyelid. The causes may be myasthenia gravis; increase in the weight of the eyelid, e.g. cyst; paralysis of the levator muscle.

28 1ml Prostigmin.

29 Immediate investigations include:

   a Visual acuity of both eyes, date and time of accident, whether protective glasses worn; type of material used and action; examination by ophthalmoscope and slit lamp; radiological examination of eye and orbit.

   b Diagnosis is made in three ways:

     i decide where point of entry is, cornea or sclera

     ii locate wound

     iii check radiograph to see if foreign body is radio-opaque.

   c Doctor advises patient as to diagnosis, treatment and prognosis. A consent form is signed. Patient's relatives contacted and informed of admission (if not accompanying patient). Surgery will be carried out at an early time. Commence systemic antibiotics. Postoperatively: read surgical notes. Maintain the nursing position that the surgeon requires. Record vital signs. When awake wash hands and face and change gown. Offer a mouthwash. Tell patient to rinse gently. Remember to approach the bed from unoperated side. Provide the radio and headphones, if required, to relieve boredom. After 24 hours, the first dressing is performed. Trolley prepared. Remove lid sutures, clean eye and observe condition of the operated eye. A doctor will probably be present, this avoids disturbing the eye too often. Note condition of all sutures and record in the nursing notes after dressing completed. Instil medication ordered. Replace dressing. Ask for guidance as to mobilization.

    Continue systemic antibiotics and continue local medications. Dark glasses when appropriate. Patient discharged when eye has settled down. Given drops and ointment to take home, instructions on how to instil them, a follow-up appointment and a letter to his GP. Advice given on not bending, stooping, lifting.

30 Photophobia: sensitivity to light.

Excessive lacrimation: constant watering of eyes.

Synechia: anterior synechia – adhesion of iris to cornea. Posterior synechia – adhesion of iris to lens.

4 The cornea and corneal grafting

Chapters 4, 5, and 6 will deal with the structures of the anterior segment of the eye (Fig. 9). (See also Figs. 1 and 2, p. 4.)

The cornea is the clear, transparent part of the front of the eye through which light rays are passed. It has five layers. From outside to inside these are:

1 Epithelium
2 Bowman's membrane
3 Substantia propria
4 Descemet's membrane
5 Endothelium.

The cornea is continuous with the sclera. The point where the cornea becomes the sclera is called the limbus. Also at the junction of the cornea and sclera is the canal of Schlemm – an important drainage channel. The cornea does not contain any blood vessels, but has a rich nerve supply from the ciliary nerves (from the ophthalmic branch of the trigeminal (5th cranial) nerve). The cornea is about 11mm in diameter and 1mm thick.

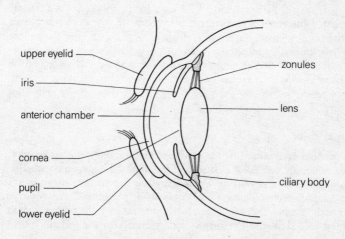

Fig. 9 Structures in the anterior segment of the eye

■ CORNEAL GRAFTS (KERATOPLASTY)

A corneal graft is the transplantation of a piece of cornea from a donor eye to the recipient in order to give the patient back sight impaired through an opacity of the cornea.

■ Reasons for corneal grafting

1 *Keratoconus*: Generalized thinning and anterior protrusion of the cornea. Keratoconus is inherited as an autosomal recessive or autosomal dominant trait.
2 *Interstitial keratitis*: Inflammation of the corneal stroma.
3 *Recurrent corneal erosion*: Past history of corneal injury which has never healed completely.
4 *Lipoid degeneration*: Fatty material is deposited in the corneal stroma; eventually vision is lost.
5 *Trauma*: If the cornea has been damaged by chemicals or molten metal.

■ Types of graft

1 Total thickness.
2 Lamellar – for superficial opacities.

■ The patient

The patient will have attended clinic for a long period (unless a trauma patient). Whatever his particular ocular condition, the doctor will have waited until the time is right to perform a corneal graft, and the patient will have known for some time that a corneal graft will be necessary to improve his sight. Before being admitted for grafting any other ocular problem should be corrected, e.g. entropion, ectropion and ingrowing lashes, as if they remain uncorrected they could damage the graft after surgery.

■ Admission

The patient is admitted to the ward usually one day prior to surgery; some hospitals will ask the patient to be admitted and await a suitable donor. Medical and nursing assessments are carried out; the patient's visual acuity recorded, local antibiotic drops to the eye and systemic antibiotic commenced. He is seen by the anaesthetist, the premedication written up and the consent form signed by the doctor and patient.

■ **The donor eye**

Because of rapid endothelial cell death the donor eye should be removed from the body within 12–24 hours of death. It is usually used within 48 hours of death, but this may vary depending on the storage medium. Swabs are taken from the conjunctival sac before the eye is removed and from the eye after it has been removed. The eye is then stored carefully until the recipient is prepared and in theatre.

The cornea should not be used if the *donor* had a history of:

Syphilis
Tuberculosis
Infective hepatitis
Poliomyelitis
Meningitis

Important note: If it is known that the donor is HIV positive the cornea should not be used.

■ **The recipient**

He is prepared for theatre according to hospital procedure. The eye has chloramphenicol eyedrops instilled, and, depending on the surgeon, mydriatics. The premedication is given and the patient transferred to theatre.

■ **Theatre**

The patient is welcomed into the anaesthetic room, details checked and a general anaesthetic given. He is placed on the table. The head block is used and arm restraints, the eye is prepared and the towels placed in position. The operating microscope will be required; it is not possible to sterilize it, so it is cleansed thoroughly and any parts which the surgeon touches have plastic pieces which fit on to the microscope and these can be sterilized. They are placed on the microscope by the surgeon who can then adjust the focusing controls to his satisfaction. There is one trolley laid up for the patient and a separate trolley with the donor eye on it and separate instruments. Thus no contamination can occur. The size of graft cut is between 5–7mm.

■ **Postoperative**

The patient is returned to the bed, made comfortable and observations checked at regular intervals. When the patient is fully awake he may be washed, changed into his own nightclothes, offered a bedpan or urinal, given an extra pillow and a drink.

Approximately 24 hours after surgery the first dressing is performed. The trolley is prepared as for the basic eye dressing. When examining the eye it should be observed for re-formation of the anterior chamber. Chloramphenicol eyedrops are instilled; either a mydriatic or miotic may be instilled depending on the condition of the eye at surgery, and the pad replaced.

If the dressing was satisfactory the patient is encouraged to mobilize fully. The eye remains padded and dark glasses are given at the doctor's discretion, and a full course of systemic antibiotics completed. The dressings are carried out three times daily using chloramphenicol eyedrops and mydriatics or miotics.

Steroid eyedrops are usually commenced postoperatively. Discharge will depend on the individual patient but is usually within 3–5 days following surgery.

■ Follow-up

The patient is reviewed regularly in clinic and the medication reduced according to the condition of the eye. The sutures are removed when the doctor is satisfied that the graft has healed and there are no complications. The sutures can be removed under general or local anaesthetic, using a microscope.

■ PRACTICE QUESTIONS

1 How many layers make up the cornea?
2 With what structure is the cornea continuous?
3 Which nerves supply the cornea?
4 What is the diameter of the cornea?
5 Define a corneal graft.
6 Give reasons for performing a corneal graft.
7 How many types of graft are there? Name them.
8 What preparation should be undertaken before grafting?
9 How long is a donor eye suitable for?
10 What swabs are taken from the donor eye?
11 Give some of the reasons why a donor eye cannot be used.
12 Give the approximate size of the graft cut.
13 How soon is the patient mobilized?
14 What complication do you think may occur after corneal grafting?

■ **Answers**

1 Five layers.
2 The sclera.
3 Ciliary nerves.
4 11mm in diameter.
5 A corneal graft is the transplantation of a piece of cornea from a donor eye to the recipient.
6 Keratoconus; interstitial keratitis, recurrent corneal erosion; lipoid degeneration; trauma.
7 Total thickness, lamellar.
8 To correct any other ocular problem.
9 Up to 48 hours after death depending on storage medium.
10 Conjunctival swabs.
11 Syphilis, TB, infective hepatitis, poliomyelitis, meningitis, HIV infection.
12 Between 5–7mm.
13 After the first dressing, 24 hours after surgery if all is well.
14 Rejection.

5 The uveal tract: care of the glaucoma patient

Figures 1 and 2, page 4, should be studied in conjunction with Figure 10 so that the anatomical features are fully understood.

■ The iris

The iris is a coloured circular membrane. This membrane is attached to the ciliary body and is behind the cornea and in front of the lens. It is an involuntary muscle with circular and radiating fibres. It has a hole in the middle referred to as the pupil. The iris is in contact with aqueous fluid (humour) on the anterior and posterior surfaces. The blood supply is from the major arterial circle of the iris supplied by the long posterior ciliary arteries.

The nerve supply is from the oculomotor (3rd cranial) nerve, and the trigeminal (5th cranial) nerve.

■ The ciliary body

This is a triangular-shaped structure attached to the scleral spur on the outside and to the ciliary muscle on the inside. The ciliary body has two structures:

a ciliary muscles which are involuntary and concerned with alteration of lens size in accommodation
b ciliary processes which secrete a watery fluid (aqueous fluid).

Aqueous fluid is a clear watery fluid formed from the blood passing through the ciliary processes and is a continuous process. Its function is to provide nutrients and oxygen to the cornea; once formed it passes into the posterior chamber between the lens and the iris through the pupil into the anterior chamber (between the iris and cornea); the aqueous circulates around the anterior chamber and drains away through the canal of Schlemm. The canal of Schlemm drains the aqueous into the venous system.

■ The choroid

This is a highly vascular pigmented coat. It is the middle layer of the three coats of the eyeball. The choroid supplies the retina with nutrients.

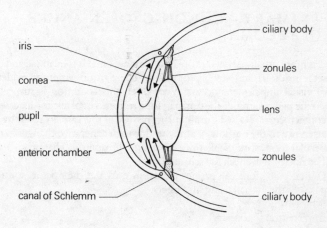

Fig. 10 Direction of aqueous flow

■ NURSING CARE OF THE GLAUCOMA PATIENT

Glaucoma may be defined as a rise in the intra-ocular pressure within the eye. It is divided into:

1 Primary: Chronic; Acute.
2 Infantile: Buphthalmos.
3 Secondary: To another condition, e.g.
    i Inflammatory: tooth abscess; tonsillitis; upper respiratory tract infection; uveitis; iritis.
    ii Intumescent lens.
    iii Dislocated lens.
    iv Following surgery: Too tight an encircling strap; anterior synechia.
    v Diabetes: Rubeosis.
    vi Retinitis pigmentosa.
    vii Perforating corneal injury.
    viii Intra-ocular tumour.
    ix Intra-ocular haemorrhage.
    x Venous occlusion.
4 Absolute – a blind, sometimes hard, painful eye.

■ PRIMARY – CHRONIC (OPEN-ANGLE GLAUCOMA)

This is more usually defined as open-angle glaucoma. It is bilateral, and the onset is insidious, and slowly progressive. There are no symptoms evident, until visual impairment occurs. Very often this condition is suspected when the person attends the optician for a routine visual test for spectacles or contact lenses. Raised intra-ocular pressure in this case is caused by an interference to the outflow of aqueous due to degenerative changes in the trabecular meshwork; Schlemm's canal; and the drainage channels.

The doctor will check the tension by:

1 Digital palpation: the patient closes his eyes and the doctor or nurse palpates the eyeball using his fingers.
2 Schiotz tonometry.
3 Applanation tonometry.
  The patient's tension may vary.
a If it remains within the normal limits, the patient's central and peripheral fields are checked (see pp. 10–12).
b If the tension is raised the patient is started on miotic eyedrops (to constrict the pupil), e.g. pilocarpine 0.5% or 1% (this should reduce the intra-ocular pressure), and followed up regularly to check that his reduced tensions are maintained. The patient will be listed to have central and peripheral fields checked, to assess how much vision has been lost.

On these miotic drops the patient is reviewed regularly and his tensions checked. If the tension stabilizes, the patient may be left to continue using miotics and is taught the importance of continuing treatment. Sometimes surgery is carried out as a prophylactic measure, i.e. to prevent the condition from worsening.

If after initial treatment with Diamox (see p. 61) and miotics the tensions are not controlled, surgery is indicated and carried out as soon as possible, after discussion with the patient.

■ Admission

The patient is admitted to the ward and a nursing assessment undertaken. He is offered help in unpacking his belongings. The tensions are recorded each day prior to surgery, and the miotic drops continued. The patient is seen by the anaesthetist.

On the day of operation the tensions are recorded and the patient prepared for theatre. The miotic drops are continued as prescribed. Premedication is given and the patient taken to the theatre.

■ Theatre

The patient is received in the anaesthetic room. It will have been decided whether the patient is for general or local anaesthetic and the appropriate method is employed. If the patient has a general anaesthetic the anaesthetist is asked to administer it as lightly as possible, as an anaesthetic raises the tension. The following procedures may be performed.

1 Trabeculectomy: A filtration operation to remove part of the trabecular meshwork to facilitate drainage.
2 Scheies operation: A drainage operation designed to drain the aqueous from the anterior chamber through a posterior scleral/corneal wound and a bleb (collection point) is formed under the conjunctiva. The aqueous is then absorbed into the collateral circulation.
3 Peripheral iridectomy (Fig. 11): A triangular piece of iris is removed to increase drainage through to the trabecular meshwork.
4 Laser iridotomy.

■ Postoperative

The patient is returned to bed and made comfortable. His observations are recorded regularly and when fully awake he is given a hands and face wash, offered a bedpan/urinal, changed into his nightclothes and sat up. He is encouraged to be up as soon as possible after the surgery.

After 24 hours the first dressing is performed. The trolley is prepared as for a first dressing, the patient made comfortable and the dressing carried out. When examining the eye during the dressing, the bleb and site of the drainage operation should be observed and also the anterior chamber to ensure it is re-formed (it will have gone flat during surgery and is re-formed with air). Following this dressings are carried out two to three

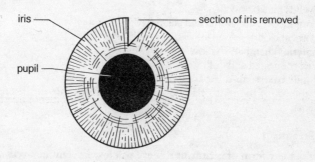

Fig. 11 A section of iris removed in peripheral iridectomy

times daily and eyedrops instilled. Mydrilate 1% is instilled to the eye twice daily even though the patient has been operated on for glaucoma. The reason is to rest the iris to avoid spasms after surgery. Chloramphenicol eyedrops are changed to Betnesol N eyedrops on the third day. The patient is seen by the doctor regularly. Visual acuity is recorded postoperatively. The patient is encouraged to participate in the administration of his eyedrops throughout his care. Additional emphasis is placed on the importance of compliance with treatment following discharge.

■ **Follow-up**

The patient is reviewed regularly and his steroid drops gradually reduced. A close check will continue to observe the patient's visual acuity, intra-ocular tension and visual fields to ensure that these do not deteriorate.

■ PRIMARY – ACUTE (CLOSED-ANGLE GLAUCOMA)

There is a sudden increase in intra-ocular pressure due to a block of the anterior chamber by the roof of the iris thus cutting off the aqueous outflow. The patient presents with a red, hard, painful, congested eye which will have come on suddenly. A visual acuity check should be attempted but inevitably the patient's vision will be reduced. He will complain of nausea, vomiting, headache and severe pain. He may be pyrexial and general collapse may be present. An objective examination of the eye will reveal:

Visual acuity diminished.
Eyelids may be swollen.
Conjunctiva: congested and chemosed.
Cornea: cloudy.
Anterior chamber: shallow.
Iris: congested and dull.
Pupil: fixed, semi-dilated and oval.

The fundus of the retina will be seen with difficulty due to the corneal oedema.

■ **Treatment**

Without any form of treatment this eye will lose its sight in a very short time. A few cases regain their sight although there is a loss of the visual field and the visual acuity will be reduced.

In clinic, immediate treatment is commenced. The tension is recorded and pilocarpine eyedrops 4% are instilled every 5 minutes to the affected eye. The regime is: every 5 minutes for 1 hour; every hour for 4 hours; then every 4 hours.

At the same time pilocarpine eyedrops 1% should be instilled 4-hourly into the unaffected eye as a prophylactic measure. A diuretic, acetazolamide (Diamox), is instituted. Initially 500mg by intravenous or intramuscular injection is given. Diamox acts by reducing the secretion of aqueous humour. After the injection, Diamox tablets are given orally 250–500mg three to four times a day or Diamox Sustets twice daily. In addition to the Diamox, Slow-K is given to replace the potassium loss. The patient is told that he will want to pass urine more frequently.

Oral glycerol 50% can be given in the clinic if the tension proves difficult to reduce; this has a hygroscopic action, i.e. draws fluid towards it. It is not very pleasant to take and can cause vomiting. It is not so widely used now. The dose is 1ml/kg body-weight.

The patient will need analgesics for his acute pain and headache, and it is advisable to give some night sedation to allow the patient a few hours' rest. During this time the patient is admitted to the ward and made comfortable. A nursing assessment is made and the relatives informed. As Diamox has been given the patient may require to pass urine frequently.

After 4–6 hours the patient's tension is re-checked. If it is down to within normal limits and the pupil constricted the medical treatment is reviewed, e.g. the strength of the pilocarpine reduced to 2% and maintained until the eye settles down.

Once this condition has stabilized, the patient has a peripheral iridectomy performed and the nursing care for this is as described under primary and chronic glaucoma. If after 12 hours the tension does not reduce, the patient is reassessed and further treatment will be according to local policy.

■ INFANTILE GLAUCOMA

This presents soon after birth or in early childhood in both eyes. In a baby or child the ocular structures are very soft and elastic, so any increase in intra-ocular tension causes the eyeball to increase in size. It is caused by an absence of the canal of Schlemm, or a blockage.

To the parents the baby may be photophobic (sensitive to light), have difficulty in locating toys, objects, etc., and some observant parents may notice an increase in cornea size. An objective examination will show:

Eyeball is larger than normal.

Eyelids: unlikely to be any change.
Cornea: enlarged and may be oedematous.
Anterior chamber: very deep.
Pupil: dilated.
Lens: pushed backwards.

■ **Treatment**

It is important to measure intra-ocular pressure. Gonioscopy and evaluation of the optic disc are important diagnostic methods.

The baby is admitted straight away and started on pilocarpine eyedrops 1% or 2% to both eyes intensively. The position regarding the baby's immediate condition and the prognosis for the future is discussed with the parents and permission sought for an examination under anaesthetic and to proceed with surgery for goniotomy. If permission is granted the examination is done as soon as possible.

The baby is prepared for theatre. He is anaesthetized and both eyes given a thorough examination and the intra-ocular pressures recorded. Remember that anaesthesia will increase the tension slightly. If surgery is decided on the eye is prepared and a goniotomy performed. The aim of this operation is to sever part of the trabecular meshwork, thereby creating drainage.

■ **Postoperative**

The baby is observed, made comfortable and given a drink. The miotic drops will be continued and the treatment governed by the tensions; the baby is discharged as soon as possible. While the baby is an inpatient, the parents are shown how to instil the drops and how to hold the baby while the drops are instilled.

■ **Prognosis**

If this condition is untreated, blindness occurs early. The eye is subject to marked stretching, and cupping of the optic disc occurs early. The earlier the condition is obvious the less favourable the prognosis. In 70–80% of cases goniotomy will control the intra-ocular pressure permanently. In these cases the long-term visual prognosis is good.

■ SECONDARY GLAUCOMA

As the name suggests it is secondary to another condition. A list of some of the conditions likely to cause secondary glaucoma is given on page 57. The patient presents with the same signs and symptoms as a patient with an acute glaucoma attack.

■ Treatment

1 Always treat the *cause* initially not the glaucoma.
2 Then measures to reduce the raised intra-ocular pressure must be taken, otherwise the patient will lose the sight of the eye, e.g. the patient may be started on Diamox. Surgical intervention may be necessary, the type of surgery depending on the cause of the secondary glaucoma.

■ ABSOLUTE GLAUCOMA

Although treatment of a patient's glaucoma is instituted, acute attacks do recur and with each attack the vision deteriorates until eventually the eye becomes blind and hard. In some patients the pain disappears but in others the eye remains extremely painful. The patient has a choice of two ways of relieving the pain which are discussed fully with the doctor.

1 He can be given a retrobulbar injection (p. 30) of alcohol: this is a small quantity of fluid injected around the optic nerve to remove the pain which may have to be repeated every three months.
2 Enucleation of the eyeball. The eye is completely removed. This is not a decision to take lightly but these patients are in such severe pain that they may welcome any form of relief. The nursing care of a patient following enucleation is discussed on page 91.

■ PRACTICE QUESTIONS

1 Name the three structures of the uveal tract.
2 What do the ciliary processes secrete?
3 What is the function of the aqueous?
4 What canal does the aqueous drain into?
5 With what does the choroid provide the retina?
6 Define glaucoma.
7 Name the two types of primary glaucoma.

 8 What is the name for infantile glaucoma?
 9 What is absolute glaucoma?
10 What general conditions will cause uveitis – secondary glaucoma?
11 What two fields' tests will the patient have recorded?
12 What do you understand by the following terms:
    a Iritis.
    b Uveitis.
    c Anterior synechia.
    d Broad iridectomy.
    e Peripheral iridectomy.
    f Bleb.
    g Cyclodialysis.
    h Diamox.
    i Pilocarpine.
    j Chemosis.
    k Goniotomy.
    l Retrobulbar injection?

■ Answers

 1 Iris, ciliary body and choroid.
 2 Aqueous fluid (humour).
 3 To provide nutrients and oxygen to the cornea.
 4 Canal of Schlemm.
 5 Nutrients.
 6 Glaucoma is a rise in intra-ocular pressure.
 7 Acute and chronic.
 8 Buphthalmos.
 9 A blind, painful hard eye.
10 Tonsillitis, tooth abscess, upper respiratory tract infection.
11 Central and peripheral.
12 *a* Inflammation of the iris.
    b Inflammation of the uveal tract to include all three structures.
    c Anterior synechia is the adherence of the iris to the posterior surface of the cornea.
    d A complete segment of iris is removed at surgery.
    e A wedge or triangular piece of iris is removed at surgery.
    f A bleb is a raised portion of conjunctiva over the drainage fistula.
    g An operation to destroy part of the ciliary body, thus reducing the secretion of aqueous.
    h A diuretic drug widely used in ophthalmology.
    i Pilocarpine is a miotic – a drug which constricts the pupil.

j Chemosis is a swollen congested conjunctiva.
k The aim of goniotomy is to sever part of the trabecular meshwork.
l An injection behind the eyeball (retrobulbar means behind the eye).

6 The lens, cataracts

The aim of this section is to:
  a give a brief description of the structure and function of the lens
  b discuss the common types of cataracts seen
  c give a guide to the nursing management of the patient with a cataract.
  The lens is a transparent bi-convex structure (Fig. 12). It sits behind the iris and is held by suspensory ligaments connected to the ciliary body (see Figs. 1 and 2, p. 4). The lens consists of a cortex (outside) and a nucleus (inside). The lens matter is made up of proteins, salts and water. In a child the lens is very soft but as age increases, the lens hardens. The lens is part of the refractive media and its function will be discussed under optics/refraction, p. 85.

■ NURSING CARE OF THE PATIENT WITH A CATARACT

A cataract is an opacity of the lens commonly associated with the ageing process. The different categories are discussed in this chapter. As the cataract increases, so the amount of vision the patient has decreases and eventually loses all sight in the eye.

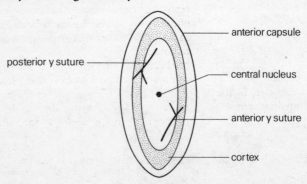

Fig. 12 The lens

■ Senile cataracts

The patient will have been seen in the outpatient department for review until it is decided that the cataract has sufficiently matured to warrant removal. He will have complained of mistiness of vision which has increased, reducing vision. He will experience great difficulty in reading and close work and this in time becomes impossible. The patient may only have light and colour perception, although colour perception itself may be altered. It will have been discussed with the patient and his consent obtained to being placed on the waiting list, bearing in mind that the majority of patients are elderly. If there is any doubt about the patient's medical history a medical opinion is sought.

■ Admission

The patient is admitted prior to surgery according to his needs. Day-case surgery is becoming more common. The patient and relatives are welcomed by the nurse and help is offered with unpacking his belongings. The layout of the locker should be explained and if the patient accepts the offer of help the nurse shows the patient where his personal items are.

He is shown the ward layout – toilet, bathroom, dayroom and telephone, and introduced to the other patients. A nursing assessment will be carried out. The patient is seen by the anaesthetist; if a general anaesthetic is not considered suitable, the patient can have the extraction performed under local anaesthetic. If any problem arises which renders the patient unfit for surgery, either a medical opinion is requested, or the surgery postponed until a later date.

Prior to surgery the visual acuity is checked and a conjunctival swab may be taken to eliminate the presence of any infection. A clear explanation should be given to the patient before the consent form is signed. Preparation for surgery will be given according to the surgeon's wishes and the requirements of the individual patient.

After the premedication has been given the ward nurse will begin to dilate the pupil of the operative eye using a mydriatic eyedrop prescribed pre-operatively by the doctor, e.g. Mydrilate 1% or phenylephrine 10%. The mydriatic used must be reversible, e.g. where the pupil can be constricted by the use of miotics. The pupil is dilated to facilitate easy removal of the lens.

■ Theatre

If cryothermy is being used the cylinder and machine should be checked prior to surgery and the cataract probes ready for use. The patient is checked in the anaesthetic room according to hospital procedure. The operative eye must be checked to ensure that maximum dilation of the pupil has been achieved. If a local anaesthetic is to be given the patient will be placed on the operating table first, positioned and made comfortable prior to the procedure.

The lens may be removed in two ways:

1 *Intracapsular extraction*: The lens is removed completely in its capsule. This may be done by using intracapsular forceps, or by using the cryothermy probe; when the machine is activated the cryo-probe freezes to the lens and the lens and capsule are removed as one.

2 *Extracapsular extraction*: The lens matter is removed but the posterior capsule is left in place.

Phacofragmentation and phacoemulsification with irrigation and aspiration are techniques which use ultrasonic vibration to remove the nucleus and cortex through a small incision. Intra-ocular lens implants are now commonly used.

■ Postoperative

The patient is returned to bed positioned comfortably (often on the unaffected side) and told he is back in the ward. His observations are taken at regular intervals. When he is fully awake, a face and hands wash is given, the patient put into his own nightclothes and a bedpan/urinal offered. He is sat up slightly then offered a drink of water. The patient is always approached on the non-operative side, to avoid his constantly turning his head to hold a conversation, etc. Also his locker should be on the non-operative side. A light breakfast is given next morning. Approximately 24 hours after surgery the first dressing is carried out.

1 Explain the procedure to the patient and make him comfortable.

2 Slide inner eye pack on to top of trolley, fix outer bag for soiled dressings.

3 Ask second nurse to remove patient's dressing while hands are washed and dried on sterile towel from pack. The dressing should be inspected before being discarded; the patient will possibly have lid sutures in place to prevent him from opening his eye under the pad. The second sterile towel is placed on the patient. In theatre an air bubble will have been injected into the anterior chamber to re-form it. This may or may not have been absorbed. This should be recorded.

The same principle applies when removing lid sutures as to any other part of the body, i.e. suture cut next to the skin and underneath pulled through.

4 The eyelids are cleansed gently with Ringer's solution, the patient being warned that his eye will water when opened to the light. The assistant is asked to shine the torch, first on the cheek and then upwards to the eye.

The eye will be red and the conjunctiva possibly chemosed (swollen). Ask the patient if he can see the light. The nurse notes the condition of all structures of the anterior segment seen and records them.

5 A mydriatic eyedrop such as Mydrilate 1% and an antibiotic one such as chloramphenicol are usually ordered. These are checked against the prescription sheet and instilled and a pad and Cartella shield applied using non-allergic tape.

Ambulation is encouraged as soon as possible after surgery. In the case of day surgery the patient will return to the hospital for the first dressing.

The dressings are changed two to three times a day and eye drops instilled as required. Those instilled will be chloramphenicol and a mydriatic, e.g. Mydrilate 1%. On the third day the drops are changed to Betnesol N and the mydriatics continued. Dark glasses are given on the third day. Discharge from hospital depends on the individual person. Prior to discharge his care will be evaluated and the visual acuity checked. It is very gratifying to see the expression of joy on the patient's face when he finds he can read a few letters on the board. In the case of the patient who does not receive a lens implant it will have been explained to him before surgery that permanent glasses cannot be given until the eye has settled down and maximum vision can be obtained. This usually takes about six weeks. Some hospitals provide their patients on discharge with a pair of +10 lens spectacles, which will help the patient to adjust to stronger lenses. It must be pointed out that these will only help the patient with distance and that everything will be magnified. Where the other eye is sighted but the patient has glasses the operative eye lens is frosted over and the patient uses one eye as he will not have binocular vision due to the removal of his cataract. Instructions on not bending, stooping, lifting, etc., are given.

■ **Follow-up**

The patient is reviewed at regular intervals and the drops gradually decreased. When the doctor is satisfied that the eye has settled down and that maximum vision has been obtained, he then tests the patient for distance and near vision and prescribes the most suitable glasses. Once the patient has had his own lens removed it is not possible for him to have bifocal glasses as he has no power of accommodation in the eye. Where the patient has normal sight in the other eye it can be suggested that he has a contact lens for the operated eye. This will provide him with binocular vision. The majority of patients are elderly, but many of them are willing to try a lens and the successful ones become quite adept with their use.

Some hospitals provide an optician's service, but for others it is not feasible; in such cases it is discussed with the patient where he should go for the provision of his glasses.

■ TRAUMATIC CATARACT

This as the name suggests is caused by an injury – either to the lens itself – perforating injury, or as a result of a blow to the eye (non-perforating injury). The lens can also be dislocated if the suspensory ligament is ruptured. It may go posteriorly into the vitreous or anteriorly into the anterior chamber. It can be treated in two ways.

Perforating injury: The wound on the lens releases lens matter into the anterior chamber. The patient *may* remain on bed rest to allow the lens substance to absorb and the pupil is dilated using mydriatic eye drops to prevent posterior synechia – adhesion of the posterior surface of the iris to the anterior surface of the lens.

If after a period of time, the lens matter remaining in the capsule remains opaque, it may need surgical intervention in the form of discission or needling.

a Non-surgical: Mydriatics are instilled regularly to keep the pupil dilated. The eye is left alone to see if the lens matter, released from the capsule, will absorb.

b Surgical – discission or needling: Under anaesthetic a needle is passed through the corneal scleral margin and the anterior part of the capsule cut to release some of the lens matter. This procedure may need to be repeated until all the cataract has been destroyed.

Postoperative care is similar to that for the patient with a senile cataract.

■ Complication

If the lens is ruptured a rise in the intra-ocular tension may occur from lens matter in the anterior chamber blocking the drainage angle.

■ CATARACTS IN CHILDREN

1 Congenital, e.g. rubella (German measles).
2 Acquired, e.g. injury.

1 Congenital: These occur in children whose mothers developed rubella in early pregnancy. Treatment is by needling as described for traumatic cataract. It is not easy to keep a baby or child in bed in unfamiliar surroundings so early discharge is the aim.

2 *Acquired*: The most common reason is a traumatic cataract from an injury. Treatment is as described under traumatic cataracts with the aim of early discharge.

■ PRACTICE QUESTIONS

1 Draw a labelled diagram of the lens.
2 Of what system is the lens a part?
3 Of what is the lens matter made up?
4 In a child is the lens soft or hard?
5 Define a cataract.
6 What do you understand by the following?
   a Mydriatics,
   b Miotics,
   c Cryotherapy,
   d Intracapsular extraction,
   e Traumatic cataract,
   f Extracapsular extraction,
   g Rubella,
   h Cartella shield,
   i Binocular vision,
   j Subluxation.
7 By what surgical method would a child with a cataract be treated?
8 What complication could occur from a traumatic cataract?
9 What signs and symptoms will a patient with a cataract experience as his vision deteriorates?

■ Answers

1 Refer to Fig. 12, p. 66.
2 Refractive media.
3 Protein, salts and water.
4 Soft.
5 A cataract is an opacity of the lens.
6 *a* Substances that dilate the pupil.
   b Substances that constrict the pupil.
   c A freezing process for cataract extraction.
   d Intracapsular extraction is the removal of the lens in its capsule.
   e A cataract that occurs after injury to the eye.

 f Extracapsular extraction is the removal of the lens matter leaving the posterior capsule behind.
 g German measles.
 h A plastic shield to protect the eye.
 i Using both eyes together.
 j Dislocation of the lens.
7 Needling.
8 A rise in the intra-ocular tension – secondary glaucoma.
9 Patients' visual acuity deteriorates, they complain of mistiness of vision which increases. Their near sight deteriorates until it is impossible to read or perform any close work. By the time their cataract is mature they may only be able to distinguish light.

7 Posterior segment of the eye, retinal detachments, refraction

This chapter covers the structures and common problems associated with the posterior segment of the eye (Fig. 13). (See also Figs. 1 and 2, p. 4.)

The posterior segment of the eyeball consists of:

a vitreous
b retina
c optic nerve.

■ THE VITREOUS

The vitreous is contained in the posterior chamber behind the lens. It is a soft transparent jelly-like mass. It has no blood supply and no nerve supply and serves to maintain the shape of the eyeball.

While the fetus is forming *in utero*, an artery called the hyaloid artery runs from the blind spot through the vitreous and joins the lens on its

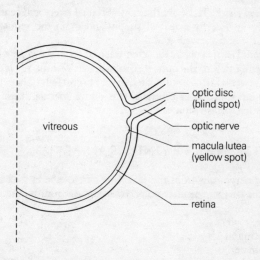

Fig. 13 Posterior segment of the eye

posterior surface. This artery is an extension of the ophthalmic artery. The function of this is to feed the lens and other structures while the eye is being formed. Before birth this shrivels up and is seen as a white string on the posterior surface of the lens in some adults.

■ THE RETINA

The retina is the innermost layer of the three coats of the eyeball. It is transparent and its colour comes from the choroidal vessels. It is made up of 10 layers. The rods and cones lie in the retina. The rods are more numerous around the periphery and are stimulated in dim light. The cones are more numerous in the centre of the retina. When the retina is viewed through the ophthalmoscope the area seen is described as the fundus. Several areas of the fundus are important:

   i optic disc
   ii retinal blood vessels
   iii macula lutea.

Optic disc: The area where the retinal nerve fibres join to become the optic nerve. The nerve head is paler than the surrounding retina. The optic disc is often referred to as the blind spot as there is no vision in this area. (No rods or cones.)

Retinal blood vessels: These are the central retinal artery and central retinal vein. They lie side by side and supply and drain the retina, entering alongside the optic nerve.

The macula: The macula lutea, often referred to as the yellow spot. It is situated temporally to the optic disc in each eye. The macula is composed mainly of cones which are stimulated in very bright light. The centre of the macula is called the fovea centralis. It is on the macula that an image is created which forms vision.

■ OPTIC NERVE (2ND CRANIAL)

The optic nerve runs from the posterior part of the eyeball backwards towards the lateral geniculate body. It has three coverings, the same three as found in the brain:

   i Dura mater
   ii Arachnoid
   iii Pia mater.

The central retinal artery and vein run alongside part of the optic nerve tract and enter and leave at the same point.

■ RETINAL DETACHMENTS

A retinal detachment is where the neural layers of the retina separate from the pigment epithelium allowing fluid to accumulate between them.

The patient presents with a history of:

a floaters

b a shadow or curtain (sometimes he will have had these symptoms for a few days or even weeks)

c flashing lights.

■ Predisposing factors

a High or moderate myopes (short-sighted people).

b Trauma.

c Tumour of choroid.

d Aphakia.

e Retinal pathology.

When the patient arrives in the ophthalmic department an accurate medical and nursing assessment is made. It should particularly note for how long the vision has been affected. It should also record which eye, what signs the patient had and he should be asked to describe where the vision is lost. The loss of vision, e.g. top half of visual field lost would indicate that the detachment had occurred on the lower part of the eye. The visual acuity is checked.

Unless there are any contra-indications the patient has mydriatic drops instilled to dilate the pupils and when the pupils are fully dilated the doctor will give both eyes a thorough examination.

A detachment co-occurs with:

a round holes

b irregular tears or holes

c horseshoe tears.

The diagnosis is explained to the patient and admission recommended.

■ Nursing care

The patient is admitted to the ward and a nursing assessment made. The patient may be positioned to allow return of the detached retina to its original position, e.g. if the lower part is detached, the patient may be nursed sitting up. During this time attention to the general comfort of the patient is important. The affected eye will be kept dilated using atropine 1% eyedrops. The remaining vision in that eye will be blurred due to the effect of the atropine.

The doctor may decide to observe the patient over a few days to see if the retina will heal without surgical intervention, or he may decide to operate as soon as possible. The patient is seen and examined by the anaesthetist for a general anaesthetic.

The visual acuity is checked, the patient is prepared for theatre and the eye is checked to make sure it is fully dilated. The patient is taken to theatre, the relevant facts are checked, the patient anaesthetized and placed on the operating table.

The eye is prepared and the towels placed in position. The detached retina may be operated on in several ways. The particular operation performed will depend on the surgeon and the position of the detachment. All surgical work is done externally over the area of detachment, the conjunctiva is cut to expose the posterior part of the eye.

1 *Encirclement*: A silicone strap is placed around the eye and pulled tight to form an indentation. It is combined with drainage of the sub-retinal fluid and scleral resection. The intra-ocular tension will be raised if the strap is pulled too tight.

2 *Silicone plomb*: This causes a local indentation and enhances indentation made by a strap.

3 *Vitreous implant*: A sterile vitreous implant which has been cultured first, or liquid silicone, air or saline may be injected into the vitreous space to aid flattening of the retina.

4 *Cryotherapy*: Negative heat (freezing) causes inflammation, therefore the structures swell and stick to the retina.

5 *Diathermy*: A positive heat is used and the same principle as cryotherapy applies.

6 *Laser or photocoagulation*: A high energy light is passed through the pupil to the retina. High temperatures are produced to form a reaction which seals the hole or tear.

7 *Drainage of sub-retinal fluid*. A small incision is made through the sclera and choroid taking care not to damage the retina and the fluid is released. This procedure is combined with any of the above.

8 *Vitrectomy*.

■ Postoperative

The patient is returned to his bed and positioned accordingly. His observations are recorded at regular intervals, and when fully awake the patient is changed into his own nightclothes, his hands and face washed, a gentle mouthwash and a bedpan/urinal offered. The surgeon will have indicated the nursing position in his surgical notes.

Approximately 24 hours after surgery the patient has the first dressing performed. This is done in exactly the same manner as described in earlier chapters. It is unlikely that there will be any lid sutures in place when examining the eye. There is likely to be marked chemosis (swelling) of the conjunctiva. The patient is asked if he can see the light. The dilation of the pupil is maintained using atropine eyedrops 1% and antibiotic eyedrops such as chloramphenicol. The eye is padded.

If the eye is settling down and the retina appears flat on examination dark glasses may be given. Dressings may be changed twice daily using atropine 1% and chloramphenicol eyedrops. The antibiotic eyedrop is changed to Betnesol N on the third day.

The patient is discharged when his eye condition is satisfactory. He will take atropine eyedrops 1% with him to maintain dilation. He is followed-up at frequent intervals. The prognosis depends on:

a How long the detachment had been present.
b How soon the eye had been operated on.
c If the macula had been involved.

No guarantee can be given that the sight lost will be returned. But surgical techniques improve and the chances increase.

■ PRACTICE QUESTIONS

1 Name three structures of the posterior segment of the eye.
2 Where is the vitreous?
3 Of the three layers of the eye which layer is the retina?
4 In the fetus, which artery runs from the blind spot through the vitreous and joins the lens on its posterior surface?
5 How many layers does the retina have?
6 Where does the colour of the retina come from?
7 Which three areas of the fundus are important?
8 What three coverings has the optic nerve?
9 What is the optic disc also called?
10 What is the macula also called?
11 The macula has most cones? True/False.
12 What is the centre of the macula called?
13 Name the two main retinal blood vessels.
14 Give the position of the optic nerve.
15 Where are the rods situated?
16 What do you understand by the following?
    a High myopes,
    b Aphakia,
    c Atropine,
    d Retinal detachment,
    e Vitreous implant,

   f Cryotherapy,
   g Diathermy,
   h Encirclement,
   i Chemosis,
   j Drainage of sub-retinal fluid.

17 What are the signs and symptoms of which a patient with retinal detachment would complain?

18 State what you understand by a retinal detachment and in what categories the holes are listed.

19 List three of the operations for retinal detachment. On what factors does this patient's prognosis depend? What predisposing factors contribute to retinal detachments?

■ **Answers**

1 Vitreous, retina, optic nerve, choroid, sclera.
2 The vitreous is contained in the posterior segment.
3 The innermost layer.
4 The hyaloid artery.
5 Ten layers.
6 The choroidal vessels.
7 The optic disc, the retinal blood vessels and the macula.
8 Dura mater, arachnoid and pia mater.
9 The blind spot.
10 The yellow spot.
11 True.
12 Fovea centralis.
13 Central retinal artery and central retinal vein.
14 The optic nerve runs from the posterior part of the eyeball backwards towards the lateral geniculate body.
15 The rods are situated at the periphery.
16 *a* Short-sighted people.
   b Patients without their natural lens in one or both eyes.
   c Atropine is a mydriatic used to dilate pupils.
   d Retinal detachment is where part of the retina is separated from the other layers of the eyes.
   e Vitreous implant may be sterile vitreous, saline or air injected into the posterior chamber to aid flattening of the retina.
   f Cryotherapy (freezing) causing inflammation; the structures swell and stick to the retina.
   g Diathermy. A positive heat is used. The structures swell and stick to the retina.

  h Encirclement is a silicone strap placed around the eye and pulled tight to form an indentation.

  i Swelling of the conjunctiva.

  j Fluid is drained from the space between the retina and the sclera.

17 Floaters, shadow, a curtain, flashing lights.

18 A retinal detachment is where all or part of the retina is separated from the other layers of the eye. Round; irregular; horseshoe.

19 *a* Encirclement; silicone plomb; vitreous implant, cryotherapy; diathermy; laser/photocoagulation; drainage of sub-retinal fluid; vitrectomy.

  b How long the detachment had been present; how soon the eye had been operated on; if the macula was involved.

  c High myopes; trauma; tumour of choroid; aphakia; retinal pathology.

8 Extra-ocular structures, squints, optics

This chapter deals with the muscles of the eye and the bony orbit in which the eye is situated. The bones of the orbit should be memorized as they will help the nurse when studying the face and head. Squints can be difficult to understand. Refer to other texts and ask to watch the orthoptist treating children.

■ THE EXTRA-OCULAR MUSCLES

There are six of these for each eye:

Four recti:	Lateral
	Medial
	Superior
	Inferior
Two oblique:	Superior
	Inferior.

These muscles are responsible for controlling the bilateral movements of the eyes in all directions. The four recti muscles and the superior oblique have their origin at the annulus of Zinn and their insertion is into the sclera. The inferior oblique has its origin in the orbital wall and its insertion is into the sclera.

■ Nerve supply

Lateral rectus	6th cranial (abducens) nerve
Medial rectus	3rd cranial (oculomotor) nerve
Superior rectus	3rd cranial (oculomotor) nerve
Inferior rectus	3rd cranial (oculomotor) nerve
Superior oblique	4th cranial (trochlear) nerve
Inferior oblique	3rd cranial (oculomotor) nerve

■ Optic pathway (Fig. 14)

The optic pathway consists of the optic nerves, the optic chiasma, the optic tracts and the lateral geniculate bodies. The pathway transmits the nerve impulses (conduction).

□ *Optic nerves*

These leave the eye at the optic disc, and run backwards and inwards for a short distance.

□ *Optic chiasma*

This is anterior to stalk of pituitary gland and is the point at which the two optic nerves meet. Fibres from the nasal half of each retina cross over at the chiasma and continue in the optic tract of the other eye.

□ *Optic tracts*

Run back towards mid-brain carrying fibres from each eye.

□ *Lateral geniculate bodies*

In mid-brain they (tracts) synapse with these bodies. Nerve fibres leaving the lateral geniculate bodies fan out as optic radiators which reach the visual area of the cerebral cortex, i.e. occipital lobe.

■ THE BONY ORBIT

The orbit is made up of bony walls on four sides forming (in comparison) a pyramid lying on its side.

Bones: Frontal   above
       Maxilla   below
       Sphenoid ⎫
       Palatine ⎬ base
       Ethmoid ⎫
       Lacrimal ⎬ medially
       Zygomatic (malar)   laterally

The orbit contains:
  Eyeball.
  The extra-ocular muscles/Tenon's capsule.
  The lacrimal gland.
  Blood vessels.
  Nerves.
  Fat.

■ Blood supply

This is from the ophthalmic artery and drainage is into the ophthalmic veins.

■ Nerve supply

This is both motor and sensory.

L   R

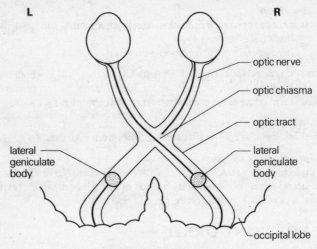

Fig. 14 Optic pathway

■ SQUINTS/REFRACTION/ ACCOMMODATION

A squint is a manifest deviation of one eye. The affected eye may deviate in any direction. The medical term is strabismus and it is due to many causes.

■ Concomitant squints – non-paralytic

The angle of deviation remains constant in all directions of gaze (Fig. 15).

a Non-accommodative: The squint is not due to any refractive error. It usually appears within the first year of life. It is possible that it is due to a congenital abnormality of some sort, e.g. abnormal nerve development or muscle insertion. It is very often hereditary.

Treatment:
Occlusion.
Orthoptic therapy.
Surgery.

b Accommodative: The error is in refraction – hypermetropia. This usually shows itself between 18 months and 4 years. Covering the eye helps (occlusion).

Treatment:
Correction of refractive error – usually successful.
Occlusion if necessary.
Sometimes necessary to resort to surgery.

■ Incomitant – paralytic

The angle of deviation is inconstant in all angles of gaze. Paralysis of the lateral rectus muscle is usually due to damage to the 6th cranial nerve (abducens).

Causes:
Cerebrovascular accident
Haemorrhage
Tumour ⎫
Inflammatory disease of central nervous system ⎬ Adult
Tumour ⎭ Child

Treatment:
Surgery if suppression has occurred – the treatment is for cosmetic reasons.

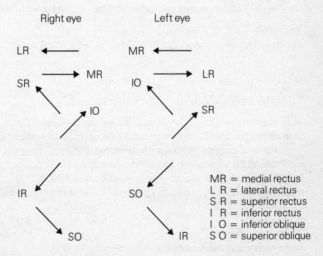

MR = medial rectus
L R = lateral rectus
S R = superior rectus
I R = inferior rectus
I O = inferior oblique
S O = superior oblique

Fig. 15 The diagram shows the six diagnostic positions of the gaze

- **Exotropia**

Less common, occurs mostly in older people. Fusion occurs for near vision but squint is manifest for distance vision.

Treatment:
Orthoptic therapy or surgery.

- **Hypertropia**

Less common. Onset usually occurs late in life. May be due to a muscle paralysis, e.g. trauma. A congenital abnormality or a complication of systemic disease which includes myasthaenia gravis (muscle complication), multiple sclerosis, thyroid disturbance.

Treatment:
Surgery.

- **Heterophoria**

A latent squint which lies dormant. Astigmatism is present and slight myopia found. If very severe, surgery is indicated.

- **Alternating squint**

One eye fixes and the other eye deviates. This alternates with both eyes.

Treatment:
Consists of resection and/or recession to strengthen and weaken muscle.

■ THE PATIENT

He is referred to the clinic by the general practitioner. The majority of referrals are for babies and children. An accurate history is obtained from the patient or parents, who may have noticed the eye turning inwards or outwards. A visual acuity is recorded if possible and the patient referred to the orthoptist for an assessment and, in conjunction with the doctor, a course of treatment is planned. This may be any of the treatments outlined earlier, for example:
Occlusion.
Orthoptic therapy.
Refraction using mydriatics.
Surgery.

■ SURGERY

The child is admitted the day before surgery. A nursing assessment is carried out and the child is seen by the anaesthetist. Parents will be with the child according to the hospital's ruling. The child is prepared for theatre, the premedication given and the child taken to theatre. Usually two muscles are involved – a resection and recession are needed but sometimes only one muscle is operated on.

The child is returned to bed and observed – when he is awake he is changed back into his nightclothes and given a drink. The eye pad is removed if he is distressed by it.

The day after surgery the eye is dressed and chloramphenicol eyedrops or ointment instilled. The doctor checks the eye and if the child's general condition is satisfactory, he is discharged.

The parents are given a follow-up appointment, a letter for their GP, ointment to take home and instructions on how to care for the eye:

1 To keep the eye clean.
2 Instruction on how to instil the ointment.
3 If an older child not to go swimming.

If the child wore glasses prior to surgery, it is for the doctor to say whether he requires the child to continue wearing them.

If the patient is an adult the same care applies both pre-operatively and postoperatively.

■ OPTICS

Light travels by rays. Distant rays are parallel but when the source is close the rays are divergent when they reach the viewer's eye. Because the pupil is a small aperture, in ophthalmology, rays farther than 6 metres are considered to be parallel.

■ Optical system of the eye

A ray of light entering the eye passes through the cornea, the aqueous, the anterior and posterior surfaces of the lens, the vitreous, to focus on the fovea centralis (centre of the macula on the retina). Because of its greater curvature, the refractive power of the cornea is greater than that of the lens. However, the cornea has no powers of accommodation; its optical function is to refract light and to be clear and uniformly curved.

■ Accommodation

To recall the anatomy (see Fig. 1, p. 4): the lens is attached by zonules to the ciliary muscle. Accommodation is alteration in the shape of the lens for near or distant vision.

Distant vision	the lens flattens.
Near vision	the lens bulges on its anterior surface due to contraction of the ciliary muscle, the zonules slacken and the lens bulges.

■ Pupil

Distant vision	the pupil is dilated to accommodate the parallel light rays (pupil dilates in dim light).
Near vision	pupil is constricted to cut out the divergent light rays (pupils constrict in bright light).

■ Convergence

The movement inwards to produce one clear retinal image.

■ Stimulation of the retina

Photo-chemical reaction between the light rays and rods and cones and nerve impulses. The pigments in the rods and cones convert the radiant energy of the light ray into nerve impulses.

Rods = Visual purple (rhodopsin)
Cones = Iodopsin

■ OCULAR ANOMALIES

■ Astigmatism

An irregular curvature of the cornea which causes eye strain and blurring of vision.

■ Myopia (Fig. 16)

Means short sighted. The eyeball is relatively too long and the parallel rays of light focus in front of the retina.

■ Hypermetropia (Fig. 17)

Means long sighted. The eyeball is relatively too short and rays of light focus behind the retina.

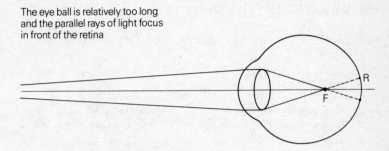

The eye ball is relatively too long and the parallel rays of light focus in front of the retina

Fig. 16 Myopia (short sight)

■ **Presbyopia**

As people reach middle age and onwards, in some patients the lens matter begins to harden and the patient has difficulty in focusing on near objects.

■ **Aphakia**

An eye without its natural lens. It loses its power of accommodation.

The treatment for the above anomalies will be glasses or contact lenses in some cases, to improve the vision.

■ **Diplopia**

Double vision. In some cases patients will complain of double vision which they find very disturbing.

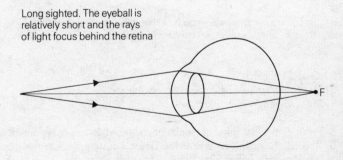

Long sighted. The eyeball is relatively short and the rays of light focus behind the retina

Fig. 17 Hypermetropia (long sight)

■ PRACTICE QUESTIONS

1 The following four are all muscles – what is their common name?
   Lateral.
   Medial.
   Superior.
   Inferior.
2 What muscles have their origin at the annulus of Zinn?
3 The following four muscles are supplied by the same nerve. Which nerve?
   Medial rectus.
   Superior rectus.
   Inferior rectus.
   Inferior oblique.
4 How many of the following do you have?
   Optic nerve.
   Optic chiasma.
   Optic tract.
   Optic radiation.
5 Name the bones that make up the orbit.
6 List the contents of the orbit.
7 Define a squint.
8 Give the medical term for a squint.
9 What is an alternating squint?
10 What advice would you give to the parents of a child aged 6 on discharge from hospital?
11 How does light travel?
12 What do you understand by accommodation?
13 What do you understand by convergence?
14 What is diplopia?
15 List the ocular anomalies you have read about.

■ Answers

1 Rectus (pl. recti)
2 The 4 recti muscles and the superior oblique.
3 3rd cranial nerve – oculomotor.
4 2; 1; 2; 2.
5 Frontal, maxilla, sphenoid, palatine, ethmoid, lacrimal, zygomatic.
6 Eyeball, the extra-ocular muscles/Tenon's capsule, the lacrimal gland, blood vessels, nerves, fat.
7 A squint is a manifest deviation of one eye.

8 Strabismus.

9 One eye fixes and the other eye deviates.

10 *a* Show parents how to instil ointment and care for the eye.

   b Give them a letter for the GP.

   c Keep the eye clean.

   d No swimming until the doctor allows.

   e Contact department if any worries.

   f To wear glasses if doctor requests this.

11 In rays.

12 Accommodation is alteration in the shape of the lens for near or distant vision.

13 The movement inwards to produce one clear retinal image.

14 Double vision.

15 Astigmatism, myopia, hypermetropia, presbyopia, aphakia.

9 Tumours and enucleation of the eye

The patient presents as:
1 A referral from the general practitioner or optician.
2 He may have secondary glaucoma from an intra-ocular tumour.
3 If it is a child the parents (or health visitor) may have noticed a white spot in the pupil and sought advice.

■ EYELIDS

Malignant : rodent ulcer.

The patient presents with an ulcer, usually of the lower lid. If it is a small ulcer, excision and biopsy under local anaesthetic. The sutures are removed after 5 days and the patient reviewed in clinic. If the ulcer is large radiotherapy is usually the treatment of choice.

■ UVEAL TRACT

(Iris, ciliary body and choroid.)
Malignant : melanoma.

The patient may present with a visual acuity defect and/or a visual field defect or as a secondary glaucoma. This tumour may appear anywhere along the uveal tract but most commonly in the choroid. The important factor here is to differentiate between a detachment of the retina, and a tumour of the choroid. The eye is dilated with mydriatic eyedrops, e.g. Mydrilate, and both eyes are examined.

The diagnosis is provisionally made and the patient is always examined independently by another consultant so that the diagnosis may be confirmed. Once the diagnosis is confirmed the doctor may request a medical check-up to exclude the presence of any secondary tumours. The diagnosis is discussed with the patient and sometimes immediate removal of the eye is recommended. While an in-patient a medical check-up will be carried out to exclude any other growth unless this has already been done. The postoperative nursing care will be discussed later in this chapter.

■ Summary

1 Sometimes immediate removal of the eye is recommended.
2 If the growth has extended into the orbit, the tissues of the orbit are removed and followed by radiotherapy.
3 If the affected eye is the only one with sight: non-surgical treatment is tried first, e.g. radiotherapy and radon seed implant.

■ RETINA

Malignant: retinoblastoma.

The patient is usually a child under the age of 5. The parents often notice that the child has a 'white' pupil and seek advice. A visual acuity is recorded if possible, an accurate history is taken from the parents, and the child is examined by the doctor. If the child will co-operate the eyes are dilated using, e.g. Mydrilate eyedrops 1% but if the child is small he may be admitted overnight and atropine eyedrops 1% instilled 4-hourly to both eyes and atropine ointment 1% at night to ensure both eyes are dilated.

The following day an examination under general anaesthetic is carried out with two consultants present to give an opinion. As it is such a major undertaking to remove a small child's eye and so distressing to the parents, the child is often referred to the larger eye hospitals. This in no way suggests that the smaller units are not correct in their diagnosis but one must always hope for a chance that the eye can be saved.

■ NURSING CARE FOR ENUCLEATIONS

The patient is admitted one or two days before surgery. The procedure and postoperative care will have been explained to the patient in the clinic, after admission and again when the consent form is signed. The patient may well bombard the nurse with questions. He should be reassured as to the artificial eye. Most departments have a patient who has had an enucleation and copes well with an artificial eye, who will come and talk to a patient about to undergo enucleation. This can be helpful as understandably patients are worried about their cosmetic appearance.

On the day of operation, the patient will be seen by the doctor and the eye marked in felt pen (by a + on the forehead over the affected eye). The patient is prepared for theatre; the anaesthetist will have visited the day before and written up the premedication. This is given and the patient taken to theatre at the appointed time.

■ **Theatre**

The patient is given a general anaesthetic, placed on the operating table, the head block is used, and before the eye is prepared both eyes are again checked, to confirm the eye for removal. The eye is prepared and the head towelled.

Enucleation   the removal of the eyeball from the orbit.
Exenteration   removal of the eye and all other structures of the orbit down to the periosteum.

If the tumour is contained within the eyeball an enucleation is carried out, but if there is evidence that the tumour has spread to the orbital tissues then an exenteration should be carried out. In theatre if it is a simple enucleation sometimes an acrylic implant with a small magnet on the anterior surface is sewn to the four recti muscles, so that when the patient has his artificial eye, this will attach to the implant and both eyes will appear to move together. If it is not possible to use an implant the socket is sutured and the artificial eye will be non-movable other than to remove it for cleansing purposes.

■ **Postoperative**

The patient is returned to bed, made comfortable and his observations recorded at regular intervals. The socket will have been packed in theatre with a pad and bandage in place, so the dressing should be observed for any bleeding or oozing.

The first postoperative day, the patient has the first dressing performed. The trolley is prepared in the same way as for any other dressing with the addition of dressing forceps and right or left sterile shells.

1 The patient has the procedure explained, is made comfortable and told that it may be a little sore while the pack is removed.
2 Slide inner pack on to trolley and fix the outer bag for the soiled dressing.
3 Ask second nurse to remove pad and bandage. The dressings nurse washes her hands and dries them on a sterile towel from the pack. The second towel is placed on the operative side of the patient. (The pad is inspected before being discarded.)
4 If the lids are stuck together they should be cleansed to remove debris and gently opened. The pack is removed using the dressing forceps, and inspected before discarding it. Any further debris on the lids is removed.
5 The socket is inspected using a torch. It will be red and chemosis (swelling) will be present. Chloramphenicol eyedrops will be instilled in the socket. If the patient is not too uncomfortable a shell is inserted.

■ Shells

These are made of glass with a tiny hole in the centre to prevent suction. They are shaped similarly to an artificial eye, available in right and left with indentations towards the nasal part. They are inserted as soon after the first dressing as possible, to maintain the shape of the socket.

The packet of shells is opened on to the dressing pack. Several sizes may be required. The shell is soaked in saline to make handling easier. The upper lid is pulled up, the shell gently inserted under the lid with the nasal indentation to the nose, the lower lid is pulled down and the shell settles in place. If the patient finds this too uncomfortable it is left until the second day, but the sooner the shell is in the socket, the better, as the shape of the socket is maintained. When the shell needs to be removed the procedure is reversed and the lower lid pulled down, a glass rod is inserted under the shell and it is lifted out.

□ *Teaching the patient how to cope with the shell*
Before the patient is discharged he must be taught how to insert and remove the shell, and how to keep it clean. Ideally the patient is taken somewhere private where he can be free from embarrassment.

Requirements:
    Large mirror.
    Tray.
    Bowl of saline.
    Sterile shells.
    Glass rods.
    Tissues.
    Towels.
The patient is seated comfortably by a table or couch and the tray set in front of him. The mirror is propped up so that he can see and the shell taken out and fresh ones made available. It will be a shock when the patient sees the socket for the first time, and naturally he will be very upset; gentle but firm persuasion is needed to get him to carry on and start practising. The socket will be tender and the patient will not be very competent at first but with demonstrations from the nurse and plenty of encouragement the patient gradually finds it easier.

During the time as an in-patient the patient is on a normal diet, up and about, the socket is dressed twice daily, and the patient is given dark glasses or, if he wears glasses normally, the enucleated eye lens is frosted over. A referral is sent to the artificial eye fitter.

When discharged the patient is given chloramphenicol eyedrops to instil into the socket, and told to contact the department if there is any discharge from the socket. He is given a follow-up appointment for clinic, and may like to continue coming to the department for help with his shell for a few days. At the same time he is encouraged to try at home, e.g. alternate days, and is given instructions on how to look after the shell.

■ The artificial eye and the eye fitter

The eye fitter usually visits the hospital when he receives the referral request. The patient is sent an appointment to attend. The fitter takes the measurements of the remaining eye, notes very carefully the colour of the iris, size of the iris and any other characteristics. The patient makes several visits where fittings are made, and is taught to handle the eye. At the final fit the patient is given instructions on how to care for the artificial eye, and before leaving to make sure it is in the correct position.

■ Follow-up

After the initial surgery and follow-up, the patient is checked at yearly intervals for recurrence in the other eye.

■ Children

The pre-operative care is the same as with the adult patient. Postoperatively the dressings and nursing care are exactly the same, but the parents are taught to cope with the shell and subsequent artificial eye. The parents will need a lot of support during this time as the shock of their child's losing an eye is severe enough, but having to see the socket and cope with the shell will be a further upset.

■ Summary

Reasons for enucleation:
1 Malignant melanoma of uveal tract.
2 Retinoblastoma.
3 Absolute glaucoma – blind hard painful eye.
4 Sympathetic ophthalmia.
5 Severe injury of the eye where neither the sight nor the eye can be saved.

■ PRACTICE QUESTIONS

1 Name the different tumours of the eye and state which structures they involve.
2 Why is a medical check carried out on a patient with a tumour of the eye?

3 What might the parents notice of a child with retinoblastoma?
4 How is a child suspected of a retinoblastoma best examined?
5 What do you understand by the following?
  a Enucleation.
  b Exenteration.
  c Shell.
  d Artificial eye.
  e Socket.
6 Any patient about to undergo enucleation will be upset and worried. What could you do to help this patient?
7 How soon should the shell be inserted postoperatively?
8 Where would you teach your patient about coping with his or her shell?
9 How would you arrange for an eye fitter?
10 Give the reasons for enucleation.

■ **Answers**

1 Rodent ulcer – eyelids, usually lower.
  Malignant melanoma – uveal tract, usually choroid.
  Retinoblastoma – retina.
2 To exclude any other growth in the body.
3 A white pupil.
4 Eyes dilated then examined under general anaesthetic.
5 *a* Enucleation is the removal of the eyeball from the orbit.
  b Exenteration is the removal of the eye and all other structures of the orbit down to the periosteum.
  c A shell is a piece of glass shaped like an artificial eye.
  d An artificial eye is the final eye that the patient receives after an enucleation. It is shaped and designed to match the natural eye.
  e The socket is the cavity left after the eye has been removed.
6 Ask a patient who has had an enucleation and has had his artificial eye fitted to visit the patient and talk to him.
7 At first dressing; if this is not possible then as soon afterwards as manageable to maintain the shape of the socket.
8 Take him/her somewhere private, free from disturbance.
9 Send a referral through the hospital channels.
10 Malignant melanoma.
  Retinoblastoma.
  Absolute glaucoma.
  Sympathetic ophthalmia.
  Severe injury of the eye.

10 Pharmacology

■ ABBREVIATIONS

Occasionally, the prescription chart may use abbreviations (basically of Latin derivation) to describe the mode by which the drug is dispensed. It is advisable always to use the full word but the abbreviations are listed in case the nurse encounters them.

Drops	Guttae
Ointments	Oc; oculentum
Tablets	Tabs.
Solutions	Sol.
Injections	Inj.

■ OPHTHALMIC PREPARATIONS

Mydriatics/cycloplegics.
Miotics.
Antibiotics.
Steroids.
Anti-viral.
Local anaesthetics.
Artificial tears.
Anti-allergic.
Miscellaneous.

■ Mydriatics/cycloplegics

These are drops which when instilled into the eye dilate the pupil

a *mydriatics* act on the pupil and cause it to dilate, and cause some paralysis of the ciliary muscle.

b *cycloplegics* cause paralysis of the ciliary muscle and this in turn dilates the pupils.

□ *Reasons for dilation of pupils*
1 To maintain dilation, e.g. inflammation.
2 To aid fundus examination, and to aid treatment of the deeper structures of the eye.

3 To improve visual acuity, e.g. cataract.
4 Investigation of errors of refraction.
5 Pre-operatively   cataract
                    retinal detachment surgery
                    examination under anaesthesia (EUA)
6 Postoperatively   to aid examination; to prevent complications.

Examples of mydriatic/cycloplegic preparations found in the eye department:

Drops
atropine 0.5% + 1% (and ointment) (this is a natural alkaloid from belladonna).
Mydrilate 1%.
homatropine 1% and 2% (similar structure to atropine but milder).
lachesine.
phenylephrine 10%.
tropicamide (Mydriacyl) 0.5% and 1%.

Sub-conjunctival injection
These are useful in severe cases of iritis when synechiae have formed.
Mydricaine No. 1   children.
Mydricaine No. 2   adults.
Atropine is not reversible and sometimes causes an allergy. The others mentioned are reversible and the patient is unlikely to be allergic to them.

■ **Miotics**

These are drops which, when instilled into the eye, constrict the pupil.
a They constrict the pupil by stimulating the parasympathetic nerve endings.
b They constrict the ciliary muscle.

□ *Reasons for constricting the pupil*
1 To reduce intra-ocular pressure in glaucoma.
2 Immediately after the lens is delivered in cataract surgery, to prevent the vitreous from coming forward.
Examples of miotics found in the eye department:

Drops
pilocarpine 1%, 2%, 3%, 4%, 5%, and 6% (and ointment).
physostigmine sulphate (eserine) 0.25%, 0.5% and 1%.
Phospholine Iodide.
Eppy 1% and 2%.
Epifrin 1% and 2%.

Ganda.
Ismelin 5%.
Isopto Carbachol.
Isopto Carpine.
Isopto Epinal 0.5% or 1%.
Prostigmin.
Simplene.
Sno Pilo.
Timoptol.
Tosmilen.
Some of these drops have the same content, e.g. pilocarpine, but are
marketed under different names.

■ Antibiotics

These are chemical substances produced by micro-organisms which have
the capacity to inhibit the growth of, and even to destroy, other micro-
organisms. They are broad spectrum antibiotics in drop and ointment
form. Some are combined with steroids.

a They are bacteriostatic.
b They are bactericidal.

□ *Uses and abuses of antibiotics*

Uses:

a Treatment of confirmed bacterial infection (after sensitivity tests).
b Prophylactic.
c Pre-operative.
d Associated with a steroid when bacterial infection is present.
e In combination to combat resistant strains.

Abuses:

a As a substitute for aseptic or antiseptic technique.
b Use leading to careless medical or nursing methods.
c Indiscriminate and unnecessary use.
d Inadequate dosage.
e Unduly prolonged treatment.
f Use without a culture report.
g Use of antagonistic combinations.
h Disturbance of biological balance.

□ *Resistance to antibiotics*

This may develop so use, either:

a short intensive course, or
b combinations of two antibiotics.

□ *Combinations of antibiotics*

1	Bactericidal + bactericidal	additive or synergistic never antagonistic
2	Bacteriostatic + bacteriostatic	additive only never synergistic never antagonistic

3	Bactericidal +
	   bacteriostatic
		antagonistic unless the
		   strain is relatively
		   resistant to the bacteri-
		   cidal member of the pair.

Examples of antibiotic drops and ointments in the eye department:

Drops	*Ointment*
Chloromycetin	Chloromycetin
Soframycin	Soframycin
Sofradex (antibiotic + steroid)	Sofradex
penicillin	
Betnesol N (antibiotic + steroid)	Betnesol N
Predsol N (antibiotic + steroid)	Predsol N
Achromycin (tetracycline)	Achromycin
Framygen	Framygen
Genticin	
Graneodin (neomycin)	
Neosporin	Polyfax

■ Antiviral drops and ointments

These are used to treat viral infections of the eye, e.g. dendritic ulcer.
Function: To combat viral infection.
Reason: To avoid further damage to the eye.
Examples of drops and ointments:

Drops	*Ointment*
Dendrid	
Herplex	
Kerecid	Kerecid
Ophthalmadine	Ophthalmadine
Vira A	Idoxene

■ Steroid drops

Function: To reduce inflammation.
Reason: To make the eye more comfortable.
Examples of drops and ointments:

Drops	*Ointment*
Betnesol	Betnesol
Betnesol N	Betnesol N
Predsol	Predsol
Predsol N	Predsol N
Cortucid	
Neo-Cortef	Framycort
Hydrocortistab	Hydrocortistab
Sofradex	Sofradex
Maxitrol	Maxitrol
Maxidex	

- **Sub-conjunctival injection**

Depo-Medrone, cortisone, Betnesol.

- **Anti-allergic**

Function: To reduce irritation.
Examples of drops and ointments:

Drops	*Ointment*
Opticrom	Opticrom
Zincfrin	
Vasocon A	

- **Artificial tears**

Function: To replace tears for dry eyes.
Examples of drops:

Isopto Alkaline
Isopto Plain
Liquifilm Tears
Tears Naturale

- **Local anaesthetics**

Function: To render eye insensitive to any procedures.
Reason: To carry out procedures or surgery.
Examples of drops:

amethocaine 0.5% + 1%
Ophthaine
Xylocaine

Local anaesthetic solutions:
lignocaine hydrochloride 2% plain or
lignocaine hydrochloride 2% + adrenaline 1:200 000

■ Miscellaneous

Staining agents: fluorescein; rose bengal.
Fluorescein is available as strips (Fluorets). Once opened fluorescein deteriorates very quickly.

Minims are single-dose containers.
Rose bengal is available in minims.

11 Blindness

Blindness may be divided into two categories:
1 The person who has always been blind.
2 The person who becomes blind.

In the first case the person has grown up adapting to his environment without vision. Very often his other well-developed special senses help him in this process of adaptation and management, assisting him to lead an independent life. Some blind people will have specially trained guide dogs to assist them in their day-to-day activities.

In the second case the person who becomes blind may initially experience a great deal of psychological trauma and practical problems in his process of adaptation. Some people, however, stress the benefit of having been sighted in helping them in their adaptation, and this is a 'tool' which the nurse may share with the newly blind person in helping him to live an independent life.

The social work department will be able to provide practical support for the newly blind person. Referral may be made to the disablement resettlement officer (DRO) or to a rehabilitation centre. Both are able to provide help for the person in his daily activities and, where necessary, with regard to retraining for work experience.

Rehabilitation centres provide practical help in a variety of ways to promote independence, to increase mobility, and offer up-to-date training courses, often involving advanced technology.

■ REGISTERED BLIND

The usual criterion for blind registration is that the person's visual acuity is 3/60 or less. The purpose of blind registration in this country is to provide practical support, with government funding, to enable blind people to live life to the full.

The following facilities are available for the blind child:
  Nursery schools
  Sunshine Homes for the Blind
  Residential nursery schools.

Some older children are sent to a vocational guidance centre at which advice and guidance can be given about work or careers, for example:

Law
Social administration
Teaching
Helping other blind people
Physiotherapy
Secretarial
Pianoforte tuning.

Training is given at special colleges. The Royal National Institute for the Blind (RNIB) provides help, information and services for the blind.

■ The blind adult

Rehabilitation centres provide opportunities for blind people to take part in sport, games, handicrafts, dancing.

Employment opportunities are promoted. There are home teachers for braille and Moon, how to read and write either system.

Facilities generally available for blind people include the following:

White sticks
Talking books
Radios
Free television licences
Guide dogs
Free travel
Free postage on cassettes for talking books (RNIB has an extensive library of cassettes)
Benefits from DHSS.

■ PARTIALLY-SIGHTED PEOPLE

These people can see 6/60 and are registered as partially sighted. They receive some of the facilities described above, such as white sticks, but generally not as much as blind people.

Advice for examination preparation

Start your preparation well in advance of the examination. Make a realistic plan of action that you will be able to achieve.

1 Decide how many hours each day you can set aside for study/revision. 2 hours daily × 5 = 10 hours weekly.

2 Make a timetable and slot in all the subjects to be studied. The length of time you allocate depends on the level of difficulty.

3 Study in the same place each day. Sit at a desk or table and have the materials you need at hand, i.e. paper, pencils, crayons, textbooks, lecture notes and a rubber. Write in pencil so that mistakes or unwanted notes can be erased (paper is expensive).

4 You must work at concentrating on your task, don't allow yourself to think of anything else so that you waste time.

5 If you are tired or upset, relax before attempting to settle.

6 Work at each of the goals you have set yourself as widely as you can.

7 Reward yourself when a goal is achieved so that you associate pleasure with studying.

8 Success is not a matter of luck but of good planning and self-discipline.

9 Learning is an active process so:

   o Study using a logical approach. Sequence the material and go from easy to more difficult concepts.

   o Don't try to learn chunks of material; skim the passage and try to understand. Underline key words or sentences. Use a dictionary.

   o Consciously recall and reinforce your memory. Commit your thoughts to paper.

   o Use mnemonics as a memory aid.

   o Ask yourself questions, apply the material, compare with management of actual patients you have nursed. Have discussions with friends/tutors.

   o Ask your tutors for help if you do not understand the relevance of a topic.

   o Learn to draw and label line drawings correctly.

   o Test yourself using past examination questions.

   o Get your relatives or friends to ask you questions.

10 Cultivate a fast reading style. Use several textbooks with your notes. Make your own notes when you have analysed the meaning of a passage. Begin to read with a question in mind and ask yourself

questions when you have read a paragraph/chapter. Read quickly then reread.

11 What you want to achieve is efficiency of study with economy of effort.

■ EXAMINATION TECHNIQUE

1 Listen to any instructions and follow them carefully. Be prepared with pens, pencils, a rubber and ruler.

2 Read the instructions on the examination paper and comply with them, i.e. start a question on a fresh page, number your questions carefully, write legibly. Note how many questions are to be attempted, how much time is allowed etc.

3 Essay questions test:
   o Knowledge
   o Comprehension
   o Application
   o Communication
   o Synthesis.

4 Read carefully all the questions on both sides of the paper, identify all parts of each question.
   o Don't be concerned that others have started to write.
   o Select the questions you feel most able to answer.
   o Tick your selection in order of sequence.
   o Analyse the setting of the question. Is the scene in hospital or the community? What is the importance of age, sex, marital/social status, environment, psychological well-being, needs of the patient in the examiner's mind? Underline these points and develop them.
   o Note the essential points that have to be made in your answer in the margin of the paper.
   o Pay attention to the weighting of each part of the question, these should help you plan the time to be spent on each part.
   o Ten minutes spent in planning is the most effective way of using the examination time.
   o When you start to write:
      Answer the parts in order of a, b, c, d
      Write legibly; be logical (first things first)
      Concentrate on the main parts; don't waffle and repeat yourself
      If a diagram is asked for make a clear line drawing and label it clearly
      Leave time at the end for reading your answers.

Remember that a good essay has an introduction, a development and a conclusion, and should be clear and concise. Remember also that each sentence requires a verb!

Further reading

Awdry, P. and Nicholls, C. S. (1985). *Cataract*. Faber and Faber, London.

Gaston, H. and Elkington, A. (1986). *Ophthalmology for Nurses*. Croom Helm, Beckenham.

Leydhecker, W. and Pitts Crick, R. (1983). *All About Glaucoma*. Questions and answers for people with glaucoma. Faber and Faber, London.

Stollery, R. (1987). *Ophthalmic Nursing*. Blackwell Scientific Publications Limited, Oxford.

Vaughan, D. and Asbury, T. (1986). *General Ophthalmology*, 11th edition. Lange Medical Publications, Los Altos, California.

Wybar, K. and Muir, K. (1984). *Ophthalmology*, 3rd edition. Baillière Tindall, London.

Index

FOR THE BEST IN PAPERBACKS, LOOK FOR THE

In every corner of the world, on every subject under the sun, Penguin represents quality and variety – the very best in publishing today.

For complete information about books available from Penguin – including Pelicans, Puffins, Peregrines and Penguin Classics – and how to order them, write to us at the appropriate address below. Please note that for copyright reasons the selection of books varies from country to country.

In the United Kingdom: Please write to *Dept E.P., Penguin Books Ltd, Harmondsworth, Middlesex, UB7 0DA*

If you have any difficulty in obtaining a title, please send your order with the correct money, plus ten per cent for postage and packaging, to *PO Box No 11, West Drayton, Middlesex*

In the United States: Please write to *Dept BA, Penguin, 299 Murray Hill Parkway, East Rutherford, New Jersey 07073*

In Canada: Please write to *Penguin Books Canada Ltd, 2801 John Street, Markham, Ontario L3R 1B4*

In Australia: Please write to the *Marketing Department, Penguin Books Australia Ltd, P.O. Box 257, Ringwood, Victoria 3134*

In New Zealand: Please write to the *Marketing Department, Penguin Books (NZ) Ltd, Private Bag, Takapuna, Auckland 9*

In India: Please write to *Penguin Overseas Ltd, 706 Eros Apartments, 56 Nehru Place, New Delhi, 110019*

In Holland: Please write to *Penguin Books Nederland B.V., Postbus 195, NL–1380AD Weesp, Netherlands*

In Germany: Please write to *Penguin Books Ltd, Friedrichstrasse 10–12, D–6000 Frankfurt Main 1, Federal Republic of Germany*

In Spain: Please write to *Longman Penguin España, Calle San Nicolas 15, E–28013 Madrid, Spain*

In France: Please write to *Penguin Books Ltd, 39 Rue de Montmorency, F-75003, Paris, France*

In Japan: Please write to *Longman Penguin Japan Co Ltd, Yamaguchi Building, 2–12–9 Kanda Jimbocho, Chiyoda-Ku, Tokyo 101, Japan*

FOR THE BEST IN PAPERBACKS, LOOK FOR THE 🐧

PENGUIN DICTIONARIES

Archaeology

Architecture

Art and Artists

Biology

Botany

Building

Business

Commerce

Computers

Curious and Interesting
  Words

Curious and Interesting
  Numbers

Decorative Arts

Design and Designers

Economics

English and European
  History

English Idioms

Fairies

French

Geography

Geology

Historical Slang

Italian

Literary Terms

Microprocessors

Modern History 1789–1945

Modern Quotations

Physical Geography

Physics

Political Quotations

Proverbs

Psychology

Quotations

Religions

Rhyming Dictionary

Saints

Sociology

Telecommunications

The Theatre

Troublesome Words

Twentieth Century History

PENGUIN HEALTH

The Prime of Your Life   Dr Miriam Stoppard

The first comprehensive, fully illustrated guide to healthy living for people aged fifty and beyond, by top medical writer and media personality, Dr Miriam Stoppard.

A Good Start   Louise Graham

Factual and practical, full of tips on providing a healthy and balanced diet for young children, *A Good Start* is essential reading for all parents.

How to Get Off Drugs   Ira Mothner and Alan Weitz

This book is a vital contribution towards combating drug addiction in Britain in the eighties. For drug abusers, their families and their friends.

Naturebirth   Danaë Brook

A pioneering work which includes suggestions on diet and health, exercises and many tips on the 'natural' way to prepare for giving birth in a joyful relaxed way.

Pregnancy   Dr Jonathan Scher and Carol Dix

Containing the most up-to-date information on pregnancy – the effects of stress, sexual intercourse, drugs, diet, late maternity and genetic disorders – this book is an invaluable and reassuring guide for prospective parents.

Care of the Dying   Richard Lamerton

It is never true that 'nothing more can be done' for the dying. This book shows us how to face death without pain, with humanity, with dignity and in peace.

PENGUIN HEALTH

Medicines: A Guide for Everybody   Peter Parish

This sixth edition of a comprehensive survey of all the medicines available over the counter or on prescription offers clear guidance for the ordinary reader as well as invaluable information for those involved in health care.

Pregnancy and Childbirth   Sheila Kitzinger

A complete and up-to-date guide to physical and emotional preparation for pregnancy – a must for all prospective parents.

The Penguin Encyclopaedia of Nutrition   John Yudkin

This book cuts through all the myths about food and diets to present the real facts clearly and simply. 'Everyone should buy one' – *Nutrition News and Notes*

The Parents' A to Z   Penelope Leach

For anyone with a child of 6 months, 6 years or 16 years, this guide to all the little problems involved in their health, growth and happiness will prove reassuring and helpful.

Jane Fonda's Workout Book

Help yourself to better looks, superb fitness and a whole new approach to health and beauty with this world-famous and fully illustrated programme of diet and exercise advice.

Alternative Medicine   Andrew Stanway

Dr Stanway provides an objective and practical guide to thirty-two alternative forms of therapy – from Acupuncture and the Alexander Technique to Macrobiotics and Yoga.

FOR THE BEST IN PAPERBACKS, LOOK FOR THE

PENGUIN REFERENCE BOOKS

The Penguin Guide to the Law

This acclaimed reference book is designed for everyday use and forms the most comprehensive handbook ever published on the law as it affects the individual.

The Penguin Medical Encyclopedia

Covers the body and mind in sickness and in health, including drugs, surgery, history, institutions, medical vocabulary and many other aspects. 'Highly commendable' – *Journal of the Institute of Health Education*

The Penguin French Dictionary

This invaluable French–English, English–French dictionary includes both the literary and dated vocabulary needed by students, and the up-to-date slang and specialized vocabulary (scientific, legal, sporting, etc) needed in everyday life. As a passport to the French language it is second to none.

A Dictionary of Literary Terms

Defines over 2,000 literary terms (including lesser known, foreign language and technical terms) explained with illustrations from literature past and present.

The Penguin Dictionary of Troublesome Words

A witty, straightforward guide to the pitfalls and hotly disputed issues in standard written English, illustrated with examples and including a glossary of grammatical terms and an appendix on punctuation.

The Concise Cambridge Italian Dictionary

Compiled by Barbara Reynolds, this work is notable for the range of examples provided to illustrate the exact meaning of Italian words and phrases. It also contains a pronunciation guide and a reference grammar.